FEMINIST
PRACTICE IN
WOMEN'S
HEALTH CARE

FEMINIST PRACTICE IN WOMEN'S HEALTH CARE

Edited by
Christine Webb

with 8 contributors

An H M + M Nursing Publication

JOHN WILEY & SONS
Chichester · New York · Brisbane · Toronto · Singapore

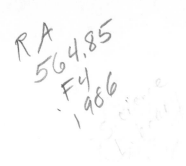

British Library Cataloguing in Publication Data:

Feminist practice in women's health care.
  1. Women's health services
  I. Webb, Christine
  362.1'98   RG12

ISBN 0 471 90995 5

Printed and bound in Great Britain

Contributors

Jane Black   WEA Tutor/Organiser, Manchester
Merryn Cooke   Student nurse and volunteer worker at Manchester Rape Crisis Line
Maggie Eisner   General practitioner in Shipley, Yorkshire
Mavis Kirkham   Hospital midwife, Sheffield
Bie Nio Ong   Sociologist, University of Liverpool
Jean Orr   Lecturer in health visiting, Dept of Nursing, University of Manchester
Mary Twomey   District nurse, Manchester
Christine Webb   Nursing Lecturer, Bristol Polytechnic
Maureen Wright   General practitioner in Bristol

Contents

Preface

As a group of women involved in women's health care as practitioners, teachers and researchers working with a feminist perspective in a variety of hospital, community and voluntary work
settings, we have written this book because we want to share
with others our thoughts about the role that feminist ideas can
play in changing health care. We believe that women want to
have a greater control over their own lives and health, and that
they therefore need information about how their bodies work,
what can go wrong with their health, what the causes of ill-health
are, what kinds of treatment are available, and how these might
work to their advantage or disadvantage. But knowledge is not
enough: if women are to have more control they will have to
negotiate the health care system, and this requires self-confidence
and a feeling of equality with professionals.

We believe that the ways of working and relating to each other
which have been built up in the women's movement can help
women to become more knowledgeable and assertive. This
requires health workers to share their knowledge and power,
and work in non-hierarchical ways both with clients and among
themselves. We hope that the ideas and experiences related in
our book will not only stimulate discussion and help us and
others to give and receive more caring, respectful and rewarding
health care, but will also be of value as a resource for students
and teachers on professional courses for nurses, doctors and social
workers, as well as women's studies and women's health courses.

CHRISTINE WEBB
January 1986

vii

Acknowledgements

I should like to thank all the contributors for their enthusiastic response to my ideas for the book, and for their dedication in carrying through the task. Several of them are not used to writing, and I very much appreciate the emotional and physical investment they made in the venture. Thanks also go to Brenda Reed for compiling the index, and to Patrick West of J Wiley & Sons for his sympathetic (but sometimes, I suspect, puzzled!) response to our ideas and efforts.

CW

1

Introduction: Women's Health Care – Setting the Scene

CHRISTINE WEBB

Health care given by women has a long tradition reaching back to the beginnings of recorded history and, without doubt, even further. Much of this history has been 'lost' as men have tried to control both the writing of history and women's activities in health and other fields, but women historians are beginning to reclaim this suppressed heritage and reveal the enormous variety and extent of women's contribution to health care.

A lost history

Documents from as far back as 300 BC prove that women were active at that time as health workers and achieved a high degree of expertise. The same evidence shows that, although men's attempts to control or stamp out this kind of women's work have a long tradition too, women have always struggled for the kind of health care they want. In 300 BC a Greek woman called Agnodice was taken before magistrates and accused of practising obstetrics and gynaecology without being formally trained. In fact, she had attended the medical classes from which women were excluded but had disguised herself as a man to avoid detection. Her arrest and trial provoked her women patients to demonstrate in her support, and they brought about a change in the law which allowed women to study medicine and to practise their skills with women patients (Marieskind 1980).

Women continued to practise medicine, and in particular midwifery, throughout Europe and to attain the highest levels of skill and responsibility, not only giving care to individual women, but also taking charge of hospitals. Anna Comnena in the 11th century was

1

the doctor in charge of a large hospital in Constantinople, and in the same century a Salerno woman, Trotula di Ruggiero, had an impressive reputation as an obstetrician. In Paris, Felicie Jacoba was brought to trial for practising medicine without a licence, and there is evidence that large numbers of women were engaged in health care as a profession in the middle ages (Versluysen 1980).

Health care given by and for women undoubtedly extended far beyond professional workers, however. Women have long been responsible for the care of others in their own homes and communities, both in health and sickness, and childbearing has until relatively recently been seen almost exclusively as women's concern. Mothers assisted their own daughters in childbirth, and skills and knowledge were passed across generations in this way, while some women specialised in midwifery and attended those outside their own family (Jordan 1978). These women were also knowledgeable about how to cope with problems in childbirth, and about methods of abortion and contraception (Ehrenreich & English 1979). In health spheres beyond reproduction, the role of women as housekeepers was highly complex and took in knowledge of herbal and other remedies to treat and prevent disease, as surviving housekeeping manuals reveal (Mitchell & Oakley 1979).

This kind of health care given by women was 'empirical', in that it was based on experimentation and observation of the effects of treatments, and was mainly learned from other women experts. 'Old wives' tales' were the fruits of this wisdom and experience which survived by oral transmission, and many tales must have had a sound basis or they would have died out as they were recognised to be incorrect. Until fairly recently, however, formal medicine and medical training were based on abstract theories, unproven and unprovable. University medical students studied Latin and the writings of Galen, Plato, Aristotle and Christian theology, and explanations of diseases were largely systems of classification based on 'humors' or 'temperaments'. Their treatments were aimed at correcting undesirable 'complexions' or moods by such means as bleeding with leeches or administering medicines made from concoctions of animal parts, accompanied by prayers or incantations (Ehrenreich & English 1979). Modern 'scientific' medicine began, according to Foucault (1973), in the 17th century when the Church consented to dead bodies being dissected so that their inner parts and workings could be observed, but even since then progress has been slow. Despite important scientific discoveries such as the 'germ theory', with all its ramifications in preventive health care, surgery and the development and use of antibiotics, 'scientific' medical practitioners still treat conditions without understanding their causes and without knowing how these treatments might work or what adverse effects they may have (Hodgkinson 1985).

Feminists have probed the history of health care and uncovered systematic attempts by the Church, state and male doctors to control women givers and receivers of care both by legal regulation and through the spread of ideas. In the middle ages the Church and state were united in England, and in 1421 the English parliament passed a law to prevent women practising medicine. Pressure to do this came from the medical profession, as had the much earlier attempts to ban Greek and French women doctors (Versluysen 1980). The reasoning behind these moves, which were designed to preserve medicine as a lucrative occupation for men, comes from Christian beliefs about the inherent evil nature and inferiority of women (Daly 1978; Ashley 1980). The Bible story tells us that Adam was made first by God, and then Eve was formed from a part of his body. Thus, the first woman was derived from and defined in relation to a man, and from then on females were seen as inferior to males. The story goes on to tell how Eve corrupted Adam and introduced sin and evil to humanity, and it sets the direction for defining women from then up to the present. Another 'founding father' of medicine, Galen, described women as 'inside-out' men, seeing men with their external genital organs as the norm and women as abnormal and therefore inferior.

Women's childbearing powers were also seen as a source of evil in Christian religion (Larner 1984). Menstruation was considered to be polluting, and so women needed to be 'cleansed' after childbirth in a 'churching' ceremony before they could take part in religious services again. Women's work as midwives, which sometimes involved delivering and disposing of dead or deformed babies and of helping women to abort unwanted pregnancies, was seen as further evidence of their inherent evilness and corruptibility (Mitchell & Oakley 1976).

These misogynistic or woman-hating ideas were used by religious and medical men in the middle ages to exclude women from medical education and organised practice, and the fact that they felt it necessary to go to such lengths suggests that women health practitioners were a powerful threat. If this were not so, why would they have needed to pass laws to exclude women?

Witches: a new stereotype?

All this evidence showing the extent of women's contribution to health care has recently been revealed by feminist historians who have proved that both formally educated and 'lay' women performed health care either as a paid occupation or as part of their housekeeping role. Although assisting with childbirth and giving care related to reproduction have always formed a major part of their contribution, women have also practised in all fields of medicine including surgery and pharmacy.

In the process of reclaiming the heritage of women's health care, however, some romantic notions have been built up which amount to a new stereotype of women (Hasted 1984). A focus on the link between women's health care and witchcraft has led to a vast over-estimation of the numbers of witches who were persecuted and killed in the middle ages and to an over-statement of their healing powers. It is impossible to be certain how many witches were executed because records are missing and incomplete, and a number of women died in prison rather than by being killed (Mitchell 1984). Also about 20 per cent of those executed were men, who were probably persecuted because of their relationship to women accused as witches.

There is little evidence in reports of trials that witches were successful healers, nor does it seem to be an anti-Church stance that led to their accusation. Indeed, many used Christian invocations to help their remedies to work and herbal remedies were not suppressed, as the survival of books on herbalism attests. The numbers of licensed doctors at the time were small and they were certainly insufficient to provide medical treatment over the whole country. Doctors preferred to work in towns, and the court in London, with its opportunities for making large profits and having a comfortable lifestyle, was a great attraction. Therefore it is unlikely that trials of witches in provincial and rural areas were at the instigation of the medical profession (Hasted 1984).

This new stereotype of witches is dangerous for a number of reasons. It paints a misleading picture of a romantic, golden age when women health workers put up extensive political resistance to attempts by the Church, state and male medical profession to control them. It portrays women as innately possessing healing skills and knowledge based on intuition and a close relationship with all that is natural and therefore good. This comes perilously close to the very religious and biologically-based definitions of 'essential femininity' which feminists set out to criticise and which see women as largely characterised by their biological functions in reproduction, as emotional rather than rational and intellectual, and as possessing 'instincts' which determine their behaviour, such as a 'maternal instinct' and 'feminine intuition'.

The new stereotype repeats these myths, and negates the hard work and intellectual effort needed by women health workers to become skilled and knowledgeable. It falls into the trap of linking the natural with the good and wholesome, and thereby obscures the fact that dirt and disease, pain and suffering, are natural but also harmful (Hasted 1984). Women's contributions to health care in the past and today are rich and far-reaching, and in our struggle to value our history we need to remain alert to possible distortions and exaggerations which could be used to corroborate already widespread negative images of women.

Medicine: a total exclusion zone?

By the 19th century, exclusion of women from formal medical practice was virtually complete. University-trained medical practitioners had managed to secure legislation not only to exclude the 'uneducated' from practice, but had also succeeded in taking over fields which they had previously shunned. Barber-surgeons and male midwives (or accoucheurs) had earlier been considered 'empirics' and inferiors because they intervened with surgical instruments, in contrast to the 'superior' forms of theoretically-based practice of physicians. However, by setting up guilds and prohibiting practice by non-members, doctors gradually achieved the power to control other forms of practice.

Control of women's health care by ideas reached new heights – or, more correctly, new depths – in the 19th century, although the empirical foundation for these ideas was absent just as it had been with the earlier theories of temperaments and vapours. The development of these ideologies is linked with the industrial revolution and the burgeoning of the newly-rich middle classes and their religious ideas (Perkin 1969). For middle class women, growing affluence brought a higher standard of living, with better standards of housing and a number of servants to run the home. The specialist role of the woman as a housekeeper was undermined and middle class women were converted into decorative symbols of their husbands' financial success. Not surprisingly, they found this very demoralising and tedious and, together with the burdens of repeated childbirth, it caused many middle class women to suffer conditions described by doctors at the time as 'neurasthenia' or 'hysteria'. Menstruation was thought to be an 'indisposition' or illness which sapped women's physical and mental energy, making it necessary for them to rest every month and avoid intellectual pursuits. Childbirth was termed 'confinement', in keeping with ideas that women were delicate and needed extensive medical care which would keep them in bed or at rest for long periods, and the menopause was considered a disease which marked the beginning of senility (Ehrenreich & English 1979).

Medical explanations of women's condition were built on notions of the female as being ruled by her reproductive functions, so that not only were her social roles as wife, mother and housekeeper a 'natural' outcome, but her whole personality and emotional and intellectual life were governed by her genital organs. Strangely enough, working class women were not susceptible to the same problems! They were seen as physically stronger and emotionally less sensitive and refined, and they did not experience the same illnesses and indispositions as middle class women. They were thus able to work 14 hours a day in factories, come home and cook, clean and service their husbands, and bear children without such suffering (Doyal 1979).

A logical extension of these ideas about female psychology and sexuality was the belief that women were totally unsuited to academic study of all kinds, but above all to medical training and practice. Education was thought to prejudice women's childbearing powers, suppress menstruation, and cause the breasts to shrink and disappear (Ehrenreich & English 1979). How much more risky it would be, therefore, if they became doctors and had to take life and death decisions when at the mercy of their emotions and reproductive functions! Medicine was an appropriate field of practice only for men, whose objectivity and rationality, and their freedom from childbearing, rendered them superior to women in this and other spheres.

'Scientific' medicine

As the 19th century gave way to the 20th, more complex explanations of sexuality were developed along the same lines by men such as Darwin and Freud. Scientific credibility was therefore added to religious and 'natural' justifications for the sexual division of labour in home-making, childrearing and health care.

Social Darwinism is based on the idea that competition within species leads to the 'survival of the fittest', or those best adapted to survival. Behaviour in humans is said to have evolved according to the same principles, so that men are on average larger, stronger and more aggressive than women because these attributes were required both for hunting animals for food and for attracting females for mating. Similarly, females have more 'nurturant' characteristics and more highly developed verbal skills than men because these qualities are needed for childrearing (Archer & Lloyd 1982). Women's rounded body shape and relative absence of body hair have developed 'to make sex sexier' for men and these features too are 'adaptive' for survival (Morris 1967). That women's bodies may have evolved in this way to provide stores of food for pregnancy and lactation is ignored in these male-centred explanations.

Twentieth century theories of child development and the role of mothers in producing psychologically healthy children draw heavily on the same ideas. The belief that 'maternal deprivation' inevitably occurs when mothers go out to work and give their children into the care of childminders or nurseries is still prevalent among child 'experts', and is used to make women feel guilty about their 'failure' as mothers and to persuade them to leave the labour market and devote themselves to their 'natural' roles (Riley 1983).

Freudian ideas are frequently used to lend support to these explanations. Even though fundamental aspects of Freud's work have been seriously challenged, his theories still underlie much of what is taught as psychology in medical and nursing schools (Doyal 1979). Freud, too, saw women's psychological functioning as an outcome of their reproductive capacity. He defined male sexuality as the dominant and 'normal' form, with female sexuality as second best and inferior. Women's psychological makeup is strongly influenced by their envy of men for having a penis, according to Freud, and women go through their whole lives trying to acquire a penis vicariously, by identifying with their fathers, having sexual relationships with men, or bearing boy children (Chodorow 1978). Women's greater tendency towards hysteria and neurotic behaviour results from their inherent psychological weakness compared with men's greater objectivity, self-control and decisiveness, in the Freudian scheme of things.

Several research studies have demonstrated that people still base their definitions of 'normal' male and female behaviour on these stereotypes, and medical workers are no different from the rest of the population in this respect. Broverman and her colleagues (1970) asked psychologists to describe a normal healthy man, a normal healthy woman, and a normal healthy person using a personality questionnaire. Stereotypically 'male' characteristics such as independence, logic ·nd adventurousness were given as attributes both of a healthy man and a healthy person, while health for a woman was seen differently. Healthy women were rated as less aggressive, more emotional and easily hurt, and more conceited than a healthy man or healthy person. Several other more recent studies have also shown that clinicians' definitions of mental health are related to traditional notions of masculinity and femininity (Teri 1982).

Research has also shown that, apart from having different standards of health for women and men, doctors see women's health problems as likely to be of a psychological nature. Experiences such as pain in labour, painful periods, pre-menstrual syndrome, menopausal symptoms and adverse effects of contraceptive pills have all been classified as psychosomatic disorders, even when perfectly sound physical explanations are available (Lennane & Lennane 1973; Birke & Gardner 1979; Laws 1983).

The division of labour in health care today

Ideas about inherent and natural differences between the sexes and their influence upon the kinds of illnesses women get and the way women respond to their life experiences also play a major role in determining which jobs health workers do. The belief that women are more suited to the nurturing, caring work of nursing and men to more technical, scientific, curative medical work are easily traced to the same origins. Even within these occupations, moreover, the stereotypes influence the distribution of women and men among jobs and specialities.

Until the last 20 years, nursing was predominantly a profession of women workers managed by women themselves. However, since the introduction of management thinking into the health services, with its emphasis on rational, objective decision-making based on cost-benefit analyses, men have increasingly taken over higher level posts in nursing. By 1980 in England, 43.8 per cent of District Nursing Officers and 50.5 per cent of Directors of schools of nursing were men, although males represented only 6.4 per cent of those qualifying as nurses in that year (Nuttall 1983). In psychiatric nursing, where men formed 29.3 per cent of qualified nurses in 1979, they occupied 75 per cent of higher level administrative posts (Pollock & West 1984).

In medicine, women find it very difficult to advance their careers because competition is intense, and they tend to fall back in the race if they take time out of their training to have children. Continuing in training while bringing up small children is also made difficult by the absence of part-time training posts and facilities for childcare. The result is that few women are found in the highest status specialities which require intensive and long training, while in areas where part-time work is possible and shiftwork is not essential women are found in greater numbers. Thus 99.1 per cent of general surgeons are men, as are over 98 per cent of neurosurgeons and plastic surgeons and 97 per cent of nephrologists and chest surgeons. Even in obstetrics and gynaecology, where more women might be expected, 87.8 per cent of specialists are men. There are no women forensic psychiatrists, general pathologists or urologists, but 32.7 per cent of child psychiatrists, 19.6 per cent of mental handicap specialists, and over 16 per cent of anaesthetists and children's surgeons are women (Dept of Health and Social Security statistics quoted by Oakley 1982). It is also clear from these figures that specialist posts involving children are more often occupied by women.

Women give and receive health care, then, in a male-dominated setting. Although the majority of both patients and health workers are women, the structures and ideas which control the system are masculine. Even where women are treated and cared for by other women, these workers are trained in and authorised by male-defined values and practices. What does this mean for women receiving health care today?

Women's experiences of health care today

Paternalism is the hallmark of much present-day health care. Professionals have a monopoly of medical knowledge and skills, and they control the situation and decide what information to divulge as well as what treatment to give. These professionals have learned a technical language which is not generally accessible to their clients, and they can use this to disguise information or to mystify instead of clarify. Because they control both the amount and style of information-giving, the medical encounter can amount to a form of deception (Lovell 1980) in which what is said is so watered down or neutralised that its meaning is distorted. A patient who is told that her cervical smear shows 'a little bit of inflammation' does not know whether this is due to a relatively harmless infection or to potentially cancerous changes in the cells.

Often the deception goes beyond disguising meaning to totally omitting information, for example about potential adverse effects of medications or the risks attached to a surgical operation. This control of information denies patients' autonomy and their right to self-direction, and makes it extremely difficult if not impossible for them to attempt to break down the hierarchical relationships which are a norm of health care. Knowledge is power, and to deny knowledge to patients is therefore to deny them the possibility of controlling their own lives and health.

For women patients, another source of oppression lies in the way their symptoms are treated but their fundamental life dissatisfactions are not placed on the agenda. Just as middle class women in the last century developed disturbances in health because their lives were meaningless and boring, so today illness may be caused by the drudgery of life as an isolated housewife, a poor relationship with a partner, or by not having enough money to keep the family warm and well-nourished. A prescription for tranquillisers will not make the problem go away. It may make life even less tolerable by provoking adverse side-effects which undermine a woman's ability to manage and it may turn her into a drug addict. It is inadequate to focus on the individual and her problems and see her condition as psychosomatic when a more appropriate term would be 'sociosomatic'. Instead of blaming her for her inability to cope, attention would then be concentrated on the social factors at the root of her dissatisfactions and her poor health, and the way would be open to different kinds of solutions.

Medical science and technology have undoubtedly made some contribution to improving our health, but the size of this positive contribution has been greatly over-estimated. Throughout history and still today the majority of diseases have social and environmental causes and the way to tackle them is therefore through preventive health measures (Doyal 1979; Townsend & Davidson 1982). It is a paradox that the relatively small positive role of science and technology has received so much praise, while the many negative results of the introduction of technology into health care receive very little attention. The dangers of the Dalkon shield (a form of intra-uterine contraceptive device or coil), depo-Provera contraceptive injections, and routine ultrasound scanning of pregnant women (Lancet 1984) emerged gradually and incompletely, for example.

Childbirth is an area where science and technology have increasingly intruded in the interests of 'safer' care, but it is hard to evaluate the overall result as beneficial. Research shows that delivery is safer when carried out by midwives, and that mother and child suffer more complications and additional interventions with each increment of technology (Jordan 1978). More inductions of labour lead to more forceps deliveries, episiotomies and Caesarian sections, and to profound dissatisfaction with or even alienation from medical treatment on the part of their victims. Childbirth has been for so long the preserve of women that male-devised and -valued technology is nowhere more out-of-place than here, and women are becoming increasingly active in campaigns to regain control over the natural process of giving birth.

Working for change

The women who have contributed to this book see their work as part of women's struggle to regain control over their own health. We all draw on our experiences in the women's movement to help us involve our patients and clients in a more truly healthy form of care. We believe that ways of relating to each other and of working which have grown out of women's groups and campaigns can form the basis of new relationships in health care.

Women's groups set up for consciousness-raising, self-help or mutual support are leaderless groups, in which nobody is dominant or has more right to speak than others. There is no hierarchy, and relationships are built on ideas of sharing and equality. Women share with each other their knowledge, experiences and feelings, so that nobody thinks that her problems are hers alone. Through this sharing, fears and anger are validated and women can begin to move towards understanding how others find themselves in similar situations and face the same dilemmas and struggles. From this shared knowledge and understanding, they can then discuss how to deal with their mutual problems and can gain new energy from other women. This consciousness-raising gives rise to the realisation that 'the personal is the political', or in other words that our problems are not unique and individual to us but are a result of the social circumstances in which we live.

Campaigning organisations often use the same principles in their struggles to gain recognition of women's particular needs or problems and to work for changes in attitudes, laws or provision of services. Leadership is often collective, with decisions being agreed by everyone after discussions in which all have the right and opportunity to put their views and nobody is given greater time or influence than anyone else. Jobs in the collective may be rotated or shared so that no woman becomes an exclusive expert, because this would inevitably give her greater power through possessing more knowledge or skills than the other women in the group. Women's groups and organisations arrange meetings in a way which makes participation possible for everyone who wants this, and provision of childcare on a shared basis is therefore essential.

By working in these ways, feminist groups and organisations challenge previous power relations and structures by adopting non-hierarchical methods and sharing knowledge and power. They see caring for each other as women and sharing feelings and problems as a fundamental part of feminism, without which achieving a particular objective – whether it be a nursery at a place of work, a change in the law relating to health care, sexual discrimination or welfare benefits, or working through a personal problem – would be meaningless.

The contributors

In writing about how we bring these ideas to our work in a variety of health-related spheres, we face up to the contradictions of being a professional or an 'expert' while at the same time trying to break down communication barriers and help other women to take control over their own lives. Being a feminist, a 'professional' worker and a person living her own life are not separable for us, and there is a continual exchange between these parts of our lives which makes it impossible to divide them up in a neat way. Personal and work experiences reinforce each other and personal, professional and political growth and development are all part of the same process.

We have come to health work and to feminism in a variety of ways and, although there are many common threads running through our separate chapters, the particular fields in which we work make our health care roles and our writing very different. We see this as a strength of the book, because it shows that feminist ideas have an important contribution to make in very diverse settings. Some of us are full-time health care workers and have written about our experiences in everyday working relationships with colleagues and clients. Others are teachers or researchers, often combining these roles with direct care-giving work. We are conscious that by no means all our clients and colleagues are feminists and that many of them may not share our ideas, and we discuss the implications of this in our chapters. In writing as women health workers principally working with women clients, we do not mean to imply that only women can give sympathetic health care, nor that only women suffer as a result of the way care is delivered at present. Our approach is feminist because it grows out of our experiences as women, and we believe that these ideas can contribute towards improving care for everyone.

The book

The history of health care for women and by women has been described in this chapter. Women have always formed the majority of health care workers, whether paid or unpaid. Throughout history women have performed nursing and medical work to earn their living, even when they were excluded by men from formal training and membership of professional organisations. Nursing and health care have also been performed by women as part of housekeeping and childrearing roles, and generations of women have passed on their accumulated wisdom as they trained younger women to take over from them. More recently, however, the rise of 'scientific medicine' has led to a takeover by predominantly male doctors of these traditional areas of women's expertise and to a consequent loss of control by women over their own lives and health.

Jane Black and Bie Nio Ong, in their chapter on health courses for women, describe their efforts to help women to regain knowledge and control over their bodies and their health. Working through the Workers' Educational Association, they organise and run courses in which women themselves plan their own programmes, with the tutor providing resources and information. Their work builds on women's demands for more control over their health and the Women and Health courses they run have often developed out of campaigns for improved facilities for women, such as a Well Woman Clinic, and in turn have led to new campaigns and further educational initiatives.

Mavis Kirkham writes of the dilemmas of women working and giving birth in the National Health Service. She talks of her role as a midwife seeking to make information available to women so that they can take responsibility and make decisions for themselves when they are pregnant and giving birth. She identifies the need for a new women's language which can replace male, obstetric language and enable women and midwives to form new concepts and communicate with each other. Mothers and midwives would then be able to give each other the mutual support which is so necessary both when working within maternity care as it is organised today and when trying to bring about changes in the system.

Mary Twomey is a district nurse who also faces dilemmas in her relationships with others at work. Although relatively more autonomous than hospital nurses, district nurses still find that doctors want to control their work. This makes it hard to work as a team and to break down hierarchies. In her relations with patients, too, it can be hard to establish equality when the district nurse objectively has more power and patients see her as 'knowing best'. Two groups of women with whom Mary works are those looking after elderly, sick or dependent people in their own homes and elderly women themselves, and she tries to help both to take more control in their own lives. The contradictions of being a feminist yet having to rely on other women carers, and the difficulties for both partners when men care for women are additional problems she encounters in her work.

Jean Orr sees the powerful potential of a feminist approach in health visiting, which is a service by women and for women. She describes how present health visiting training courses reinforce stereotyped views of women principally as mothers and rarely as people in their own right, and how they focus on individual problems rather than examining the social influences which give rise to women's isolation and depression, and to violence in the family. She believes that the disciplines of medicine and sociology have excluded women from study and have seen women as secondary to men, so that masculine behaviour becomes 'normal' and feminine behaviour 'abnormal' or 'deviant'. Like Mavis Kirkham, she identifies a need for a female language and ways of thinking about women's lives and health, which would enable health visitors and the women they seek to help to talk about issues on their own terms and work together towards solutions.

Christine Webb writes about her research work with gynaecology patients and nurses. Through her studies of women having a hysterectomy and her own experiences as a gynaecology patient, she was led to ask why nurses – the majority of whom are themselves women – do not identify with and give more support to gynaecology patients. She found that the dominating ideas of male doctors, which define women as emotional and manipulating, took greater precedence in nurses' thinking than the experiences and feelings they shared with their women patients. When interviewing hysterectomy patients, she found that they often lacked the most basic information about their operation, treatment and likely progress, and so she turned her research interviews into an exchange of information with the women. She believes that nurses, as women, are in a unique position to challenge negative attitudes towards women and to help women patients to gain information. In this way, the amount of control women have over their lives and health can grow, and feminist ideas can be a powerful way to achieve change.

Maggie Eisner and Maureen Wright describe the dilemmas over power and authority they face as doctors and feminists. Different levels of work are possible as a general practitioner, and they discuss their relationships with other workers in the health centres where they work, their work with those who consult them, and their wider political work in women's groups and organisations. Despite the struggles involved in working as a feminist within a male-defined structure, they both gain deep satisfaction and are greatly challenged by their individual work with women patients.

Merryn Cooke writes about her counselling work with women, in which she tries to form equal relationships, to help women understand their own feelings and to allow themselves time to work through these. She hopes through her counselling to offer a wide range of choices and alternatives to women and to support them as they struggle towards the changes they choose for themselves. She describes the arrangements necessary for effective counselling work in order to give support to counsellors and ensure that they know and trust each other. She believes that her counselling needs to be done in combination with wider political and educational work – around struggles to change male definitions of rape, for example – and not in isolation.

Bie Nio Ong is a feminist researcher who writes about her study of women who abused their children. She challenges explanations of child abuse which place all responsibility on individual women and do not question how women are defined and the kinds of roles they are allocated in society. In her research she began to develop ways of helping women to share their experiences of violence and abuse with other women and, like Christine Webb, she sees research with women as a two-way exchange in which the researcher gives to the women she interviews as well as gathering information from them. As a feminist and a mother herself, she had to confront the 'vast spaces' between her own ideas about childcare and those of the women she worked with. She believes that those working with abusing women need to reconsider their own definitions of motherhood if they are to understand the situations in which their clients find themselves.

The shared ideas, working methods, dilemmas and contradictions we face as feminists working in women's health care are brought together in the concluding chapter, where we re-affirm our belief that sharing knowledge and experiences, breaking down unequal working relationships, and recognising the struggles and strengths we share as women can be powerful forces for change in health care. We have written this book because we believe that, by challenging male definitions of femininity and health, by working together in these different ways, and by giving each other support in our struggles, women can take back control over our own bodies and our own health.

References

Archer J & Lloyd B (1982) *Sex and Gender.* Harmondsworth : Penguin

Ashley J A (1980) Power in structured misogyny: implications for the politics of care. *Advances in Nursing Science,* **2** (3), 3–22

Birke L & Gardner K (1979) *Why Suffer? Periods and their Problems.* London: Virago

Broverman IK, Broverman DM, Clarkson FE, Rosenkrantz PS & Vogen SR (1970) Sex role stereotypes and clinical judgements of mental health. *Journal of Consulting and Clinical Psychology,* **34**, 1–7

Chodorow N (1978) *The Reproduction of Mothering. Psychoanalysis and the Sociology of Gender.* Berkeley: University of California Press

Daly M (1978) *Gyn/Ecology: the Metaethics of Radical Feminism.* Boston: Beacon Press

Doyal L (1979) *The Political Economy of Health.* London: Pluto Press

Ehrenreich B & English D (1979) *For Her Own Good. 100 Years of the Experts' Advice to Women.* London: Pluto Press

Foucault M (1973) *The Birth of the Clinic.* London: Tavistock Publications

Hasted R (1984) The new myth of the witch. *Trouble & Strife,* **2**, 10–17

Hodgkinson N (1985) The bitterest of pills to have to swallow. *The Guardian,* 6 February

Jordan B (1978) *Birth in Four Cultures.* Quebec: Eden Press

Lancet (1984) Editorial: Diagnostic ultrasound in pregnancy. *Lancet,* **ii**, 201–202

Larner C (1981) *Enemies of God: the Witch-hunt in Scotland.* London: Chatto & Windus

Laws S (1983) The sexual politics of premenstrual tension. *Women's Studies International Forum,* **6**, 1, 19–31

Lennane KJ & Lennane MB (1973) Alleged psychogenic disorders in women – a possible manifestation of sexual prejudice. *New England Journal of Medicine,* **288** (6), 288–292

Lovell MC (1980) The politics of medical deception: challenging the trajectory of history. *Advances in Nursing Science,* **2** (3), 73–86

Marieskind HI (1980) *Women in the Health System. Patients, Providers, and Programs.* St Louis: CV Mosby

Mitchell L (1984) Enemies of God or victims of patriarchy? *Trouble & Strife,* **2**, 18–20

Mitchell J & Oakley A eds (1976) *The Rights and Wrongs of Women.* Harmondsworth: Penguin

Morris D (1967) *The Naked Ape*. London: Jonathan Cape
Nuttall P (1983) Male takeover or female giveaway? *Nursing Times*, 12
    January, 10–11
Oakley A (1982) *Subject Women*. London: Fontana
Perkin H (1969) *The Origins of Modern English Society 1780–1880*. London:
    Routledge & Kegan Paul
Riley D (1983) *War in the Nursery. Theories of the Child and Mother*.
    London: Virago
Teri L (1982) Effects of sex and sex-role style on clinical judgement. *Sex
    Roles*, **8** (6), 639–649
Townsend P & Davidson N (1982) *Inequalities in Health*. Hardmonds-
    worth: Penguin
Versluysen MC (1980) Old wives' tales? Women healers in English
    history. In Davies C ed *Rewriting Nursing History*, London:
    Croom Helm

2

Women and Health Courses: Our Bodies, Our Business

JANE BLACK · BIE NIO ONG

About the Authors

Jane Black

I first began to understand fully the links between women's health and women's self-confidence and control when I worked as a volunteer counsellor at a Women's Information Centre in Montreal, Canada in 1975. The Centre's work – individual advice and group discussions – was of enormous value to the women it served.

Later I worked in London for Gingerbread, which is a national association for single-parent families, the majority of whom are women. I helped to set up local self-help groups, and gave practical support to existing groups. I saw many examples of what can be achieved collectively to overcome the difficulties and isolation of single parenthood, including childcare schemes, social activities, mutual support, welfare rights advice, and so on.

Since moving back to my home town of Manchester in 1978, I have worked for the Workers' Educational Association. I began as a development worker, organising courses based in the inner city, focusing on issues such as health and working mainly with black groups. Later, I became responsible for teaching and organising women's education in the North Western District.

In the kind of job I do there is a very thin line between 'work' and what I would choose to do out of interest and commitment. Outside work, I have been a member of a feminist self-help therapy group for two years, and have been active in various other campaigns on women's issues in the community and in my trade union. I am also involved in producing a Jewish feminist magazine called Shifra.

Bie Nio Ong

I am a sociologist specialising in research on women, both in the First and Third Worlds. My work focuses on health and medicine, and at the moment I am

19

carrying out a project concerned with care in the community. I am attached to the Universities of Liverpool and Hull, and combine research with teaching. As I live in Liverpool, my political commitments are very much bound up with the problems of the city and I am involved in a campaign to safeguard services for women, in particular the Women's Hospital which is threatened with closure. I have a son and a daughter.

Within women's struggles of the last decade, the women's health movement has played a crucially important role (Doyal 1983). Our word play on the well-known book *Our Bodies, Ourselves* (Phillips & Rakusen 1979) – which is one of the landmarks in the women's health movement – is closely connected with those struggles. We chose this title to stress that restoring the feeling of being in touch with our bodies and recapturing control through gaining greater knowledge are prime concerns of Women and Health work. In this chapter we focus on the contribution made by Women and Health courses towards this goal. We first discuss the historical development by the Workers' Educational Association (WEA) of Women's Studies courses in the North West of England and we then outline the overall aims and perspectives of this work. This is followed by a description of different methods and approaches, and discussion of some of the problems encountered. We have included two specific examples of topics often discussed in the courses. We go on to describe the ways in which this work is received by local branches of the Workers' Educational Association, and the links between the courses and both personal and collective action. Finally, we pose the question of how much we can realistically achieve in the courses and, against the background of progress up to the present, we shall outline some ways forward.

Women and health courses in the North-West

Both nationally and locally the Workers' Educational Association has played an important role in promoting Women's Studies. In the North West, Women and Health courses, in particular, attract large attendances and succeed in recruiting students who would not normally attend an adult education class.

The first request for a Women and Health course in Manchester came in 1979 from a local women's group in Levenshulme who were concerned about health care provision for local women. The WEA, a national voluntary body providing adult education and registered as a charity with no party political or sectarian ties, had a strong presence in the Levenshulme area with their Trade Union and Basic Education/WEA project (TUBE 1981). The organisation was able to help to set up an eight week course with the women's group and on this basis a successful campaign was built up for a Well Women Clinic, the first one in Manchester.

Over the last four years a growing number of women and health courses have been established in various forms including evening classes, day-time classes with child care, and one-day schools, in a variety of places such as community centres, health centres and local schools, and in co-ordination with mother-and-toddler groups and groups of Asian and Afro-Caribbean women. Similar developments have taken place elsewhere and have grown into a Women's Health Shop in Edinburgh and the London-based Women's Health Information Centre. Nationally, there has been a growing interest in women's health issues as may be seen from the increasing number of publications on the subject, the growth of Well Women Clinics and the Well Women TV programmes.

The reasons why the NW District of the WEA has made the provision of women and health courses a main area of work are two-fold: firstly, the overwhelming demand for those courses in the last four years and, secondly, the recognition that certain regions of the country are deprived in terms of overall health of the population and allocation of resources. NW England is one of these regions and very little work has been done in relation to women's health in these deprived areas. From experience of Women and Health courses it became clear that there was a great unmet need for basic health education for women on a range of issues, and an expansion of the network of courses seemed to be needed to tackle the evident demand for more knowledge about health services and health problems.

The majority of users of the health service are women. This is partly because there are more women than men in the population and partly because women consult on behalf of those they care for: children, the sick and elderly. In addition, women are subject to 'medicalisation', that is they are classed as patients during natural physiological processes such as pregnancy and childbirth (Oakley 1980). Not only is there much evidence that women cannot afford to be sick (Leeson & Gray 1979), but many women also find it difficult to explain fully to their doctors how they feel (Roberts 1980). Health education for women, therefore, can have the effect of improving the relationship between a woman and her doctors, as well as giving the woman far greater overall knowledge of her health.

The North West is a region hard hit by unemployment, and in some pockets of Manchester this is as high as 30%. There is a clear relationship between unemployment and health (Unemployment and Health Study Group 1983) and this affects women too, either because they are unemployed workers themselves, or because they have to cope with the effects of unemployment within the family (Graham 1984).

Overall, greater ill-health, poor access to existing health services, and the fact that the services themselves might be difficult to cope with combine to produce a picture of general deprivation and poor levels of health care.

Within this context, health education is seen as increasingly important in improving standards of health and the WEA can play a powerful role in this field, precisely because of its organisational structure. The WEA is democratically organised, which means that by attending a class a student becomes a WEA member and can put her or his views forward within the local branches which decide what classes are run in the future; it is able, therefore, genuinely to reflect the wishes of class members in its organisation and policy-making, and this aspect is very important in Women and Health courses. Women can participate in decisionmaking on the priorities in their courses and are thus able to determine which needs are to be met: in this way they have a great influence upon the content of the sessions. The courses not only provide them with knowledge in their daily life, but also serve as a framework for promoting change and can take health education out of the individualised sphere of 'looking after yourself'.

In the North West, all these influences have led to the continuing expansion of Women and Health courses and have also contributed to the development of women's studies generally and the appointment in 1982 of a Specialist Tutor/Organiser responsible for Women's Studies, in the person of Jane Black.

Aims and objectives

The aims of Women's Studies courses generally and Women and Health work in particular are fundamentally similar. In parallel with Mary Evans' article in *Feminist Review* (Evans 1982), we argue that our work in the Women and Health Courses challenges dominating masculine ideas, in particular those of the medical profession. Secondly, we propose a radical change in how we see the world – we want to define health and illness from the perspective of women's own experiences and open up alternatives in order to take control over knowledge. Thus, we want to challenge the 'natural order' where women are passive consumers of health services and are subject to the oppression which is built into medical knowledge, with its sexist, racist and class bound notions about femalehood. Women's health knowledge has become devalued with the rise of scientific medicine, as Christine Webb outlines in the Introduction. In stating our first two objectives as challenging ideas and, in particular, the ways in which women are perceived in medical thinking, we want to change medical knowledge for both women and professionals.

Thirdly, as an extension of the second point, we ask questions about why women become ill. We make connections between women's roles in society (carer, worker, mother, wife, and so on) and patterns of health and illness among women. Thus, we hope to break away from individualistic explanations of ill-health.

Working methods

In Women and Health courses, women are encouraged to work as a group and to use the information disseminated in the group not just for individual gain in self-confidence but to share and develop knowledge through collective discussion. We feel that it is important for women to understand why they have lost touch with their own knowledge and are therefore not relying on their own judgements. In group discussions, women can recapture medical knowledge and relate it to their own experiences, self-image and concepts of health and illness. Most importantly, they can share. Our society individualises people and, by cutting them off from each other, makes them powerless. By sharing, we can go beyond individual experiences, begin to see the more general patterns of health and illness, and relate these to women's role in society and to how we are oppressed by being kept ignorant as a group. These shared insights, often resulting in shared anger, serve as a catalyst for change – we learn because we want to change. This may be individual change, through learning how to cope with our own bodies, how to handle encounters with medical professionals, or where to go for advice and help, or it may be collective action through campaigning for better facilities in our own areas or for a well women clinic, for example. This differs from the kind of health education which puts the emphasis on individual responsibility for correcting an 'unhealthy' lifestyle. The main focus in Women and Health courses is on active participation of women, on encouraging a process of self-analysis, and on analysis of wider social processes which can provide a stimulus for change.

Teaching is informal, with discussion and sharing of experiences rather than a formal lecture, because a conventional hierarchical relationship between student and teacher is unable to incorporate the notion of change as we see it. A main aim we have as tutors is to break down the barriers imposed on us by traditional teaching practices, and our emphasis on sharing experiences means that we, as tutors, also take part in that process. We therefore have to be prepared to 'open up' and become personally involved, and the implications of this for a learning process are many. There are no 'active/passive' or 'giver/receiver' relationships, participation is stimulated, and responsibility is shared through discussion, verbal and non-verbal activities. The tutor acts as facilitator and guide and the boundaries between learning and therapy are fluid.

In practice, these changes mean that from the start the group has to take responsibility for the course in the sense of determining the content of the series. There is no 'typical' Women and Health course; instead there is a flexible model which can be adapted to the needs of a particular group. The choice of topics differs from course to course but, however many topics are included, care is taken to provide some form of continuity. This is often guaranteed in the person of one tutor, even if there are outside speakers who come in for specific sessions. In the first session of the course, the women who have come are asked to introduce themselves and to voice their needs. Only after the discussion of what every group member wants to get out of the course is the final programme of sessions agreed. It often happens that many of the topics that a tutor has prepared or proposed are included, but sometimes the emphasis is changed or new topics are added and others discarded.

Many courses have included practical discussions on such issues as contraception, pregnancy, food, and so on, revealing a tremendous need for basic health education geared towards women. Topics such as pre-menstrual tension, cystitis, the menopause, depression and infertility come up as well, and these also are subjects which are rarely discussed in a group situation. Women may also feel inhibited about talking at length to their GPs about this kind of problem. Discussions about attitudes towards health and health care in our society and their effects on women also take place.

The tutor takes responsibility for providing information for all sessions. Because sessions are to a great extent controlled by students both in content and in form, they are able to identify strongly with the issues discussed. This sometimes means that women are able to discuss experiences and feelings they have not hitherto found it easy to disclose. For some women this can be a painful experience that is not always anticipated by themselves or understood by others in the group. In these situations the tutor provides space and support for the distressed individual but at the same time places her experience within a wider perspective by sharing it with the group, and showing how it links with women's position in society. It is here that the boundaries between teaching and therapy cannot be clearly drawn. While we do not offer individual psychotherapy, we consider that the therapeutic aspect of our work is, in principle, the same as the goals of adult education, namely facilitating personal development and, therefore, that blurring these boundaries is an inevitable and positive aspect of the course.

There is a commitment to encouraging students to develop a clearer idea of their own health choices and more confidence in approaching the health services. In line with this commitment, information is presented in accessible form, closely linked to women's own experiences. Gaining information enhances the women's self-confidence, because they can then better understand their own bodies and what happens to them, and relate this to wider processes in society, to their own position as women, and their relationships with others. This self-confidence is important to women individually when they have to cope with illness, and when they encounter medical personnel. Many of us feel overwhelmed by scientific knowledge and jargon, so understanding our own bodies and feeling able to rely on our own observations can help to demystify medicine and its practitioners. The process of understanding and validating our own feelings is crucial in gaining more control and in facing professionals as informed and confident people who can participate in decisions made about our health care.

Even if there is no 'typical' course, certain ingredients are always present and an informal atmosphere is considered to be crucially important in attracting women and encouraging them to continue the courses. To this end, attention is paid to details such as arranging seating in circles, with the possibility of working in smaller sub-groups, providing coffee and tea, and having time before or after the sessions to talk more with each other. For day-time classes, the provision of child care is essential in order to attract women who have the greatest need, especially those with little money, poor access to resources, and having domestic responsibilities. This is in line with WEA national policy which recognises the importance of child care provisions (WEA 1982).

To illustrate how these principles are put into practice, we shall describe two examples of topics much discussed on courses.

Mental health

A session on mental health, often called 'Stresses and Strains' always attracts a great deal of interest. It is obviously of central importance to many women and we try to emphasise this in the short handouts we use to introduce such a session. One example reads as follows:

> All of us experience stress at some time in our life. Sometimes you feel you can cope with stress, sometimes not. This depends on all sorts of factors, which are related to family life, work, social situation, physical health etc. However, most women see stress as an individual problem, as if they themselves are the person to be blamed for feeling tense or depressed. Why is this?
>
> Society's approach, and in particular a medical approach, tends to define stress in women differently from stress in men. Firstly, stress in men is often taken more seriously and is seen as resulting from work. For men, stress is frequently defined more in physical terms: for example, they get ulcers or heart disease. Secondly, stress in women is more often seen as a problem within themselves, as a personality problem, and more often defined as depression or mental illness. This difference is oppressive for women because:
>
> 1   women's work is equally as stressful as men's, often even more so because women may carry the double burden of a job and domestic responsibilities,
>
> 2   real physical illness in women is often explained as 'neurosis' and inadequately treated with tranquillisers, and
>
> 3   women are stigmatised as being naturally weaker, less able to cope and less able to carry responsibility.
>
> How do you feel about these things, and what alternatives do we have?

This handout raises many issues for discussion, from individual experiences to those shared by group members, and at the same time looks at how society and medicine see women's 'nature' and women's role. Many women become angry about what has happened to them and to other women in the group, but this anger is soon turned into the question 'But what can we do?'. The group might discuss solutions in individual cases, such as that of a woman who wanted to solve her addiction to Valium, or look at alternative therapies and local agencies that could help, or talk more generally about how to convince a doctor that one does not automatically want tranquillisers as a first line of treatment. We might consider how to make oneself stronger in order to confront others and stand up for oneself, and this might lead to discussions about assertiveness, confidence and relaxation. We have also done relaxation exercises in the group under the tutor's guidance. These can be pleasant in themselves but may also help to teach women how to recognise areas of tension within themselves.

Depending upon the wishes of the members, the session might focus mainly on talking about the problem of stress, either as a whole group or in smaller groups. The women might then proceed to work out strategies for change on an individual and a group level. Some courses have opted for more exercises, or for working out how to set up an assertiveness training group. The fact that there are several ways to approach this topic, and different strategies for tackling the problem, shows how effective sharing responsibility in the group and adapting the courses to individual and group needs can be.

Premenstrual tension and painful periods

Many women suffer from premenstrual tension (PMT) or painful periods and often their initial response when this topic is raised is one of sheer relief that here is an opportunity to talk about how they feel. At the same time, PMT and menstruation are seen as negative experiences, and we try to present them as natural, healthy processes in the first instance and not as an experience we dislike or find shameful. Again, we might use a short handout and open up the discussion with questions that encourage women to share their experiences:

> 1 At what age did you begin to menstruate? How did you first learn about it. Did you feel adequately prepared?
> 2 When you learned about menstruation, did you know 'how babies were made?' Did you understand the link between sex and reproduction? Did your attitude towards boys change?
> 3 Did your attitude towards yourself change? What were your feelings?
> 4 Are you aware of any physical or emotional changes during the menstrual cycle?
> 5 Have you found any useful ways of coping with PMT or period pain?

The negative image that menstruation has in our culture, and in many others, has helped to shape women's experiences (Laws 1983), and in looking at this subject, we attempt once and for all to put aside the notion of menstruation as a 'curse', as a burden for women to bear silently. Discussion can develop in several ways, depending on the interests and concerns of women in the group; for example, some groups will focus on premenstrual tension, others on painful periods.

The tutor will bring along plenty of factual information about the workings of the menstrual cycle, with diagrams and handouts and, perhaps, a pelvic model. We find that women really value the chance to gain basic information about their cycle and how it works, and are far less intimidated in the safe and informal atmosphere of the course. This discussion also links well with other parts of the course, for instance those sessions dealing with contraception and fertility.

In discussion, we might begin to explore the possible causes of premenstrual tension and dysmenorrhoea, and to examine potential remedies. There are no 'right' or 'wrong' answers in this area, just a range of options to try. It is often through trial and error, and by sharing experiences with other women, that a woman will be able to discover what the most helpful solutions are for her, which might include changes in diet, exercise, practical relaxation, herbal remedies and vitamins.

These practical concerns are closely linked with discussions of society's attitudes towards menstruation which, as we have indicated, can be at the root of many women's negative experiences. We attempt to translate these abstract ideas into practical and emotional support for individual women, and respect for how they experience their own problems.

In one town where a successful Women and Health Course had been held, one woman decided to try and start a PMT self-help group and, after discussion with the course tutor and other women, began to feel confident enough to do so. Two years later the group still meets regularly, and it has provided a way for many local women to develop their own knowledge and control of this aspect of their health.

Dilemmas and problems

Because of the experimental nature of the courses, it was perhaps inevitable that these gave rise to several problems. In 1982, three tutors felt the need to support each other in a structured manner and so held regular meetings to discuss three difficult areas.

Content of the courses   All three tutors had different course outlines because the needs of their groups differed according to age structure, area, local facilities, and so on, yet were able to discuss the political direction of their work, how they put that into practice, and how they could relate to other activities or groups in the area and to the women's own political directions. They used the term 'political' here to indicate the wish to take control over one's own life and to change things, and not in the sense of 'party political'. They were also able to co-ordinate the use of certain teaching materials, films, and so on, within the group of tutors working together.

Teaching methods   So-called democratic, action-oriented teaching requires different approaches which are not always shared by students themselves. Certain students expect a more formal teacher/student relationship and are not ready to accept the responsibility needed in our approach. This has led to conflict in a number of instances where the students accused a tutor of not 'disciplining' others in the group, which often meant that they wanted the tutor to stop the more 'talkative' women speaking of their own experiences. We have to admit that this causes real dilemmas, as some women also use the courses to discharge their emotions and thereby allow the others very little space. The question remains of how to control this kind of group interaction in constructive ways.

Our personal involvement   The overall aims of the courses are basically feminist but we are confronted with the dilemma which is discussed by Angela McRobbie in 1982. She states that feminists have to come to terms with the 'vast spaces' between themselves and other women. The fact that we are working with women does not automatically mean that we share the same world views, and this consideration has important implications. In our courses we certainly do not want to 'convert' anyone. At the same time, we feel that we have to be quite explicit about our own stance, without exploiting the tutor/student relationship. Thus we have to be prepared to discuss differences as equals, and to learn from women in the group. Sometimes we become engaged in heated debates when the group is discussing their different experiences of the same events, for example, whether childbirth is safer in hospital or at home, and everyone puts forward her own opinions.

A broader political problem is that Women and Health courses are run by people outside the structure of the NHS, while at the same time they want to influence the service. There is a paradox between encouraging women to use the health service more fully, while at the same time criticising that service. The answer lies in the explicit aim of the courses, which is to increase women's assertiveness to demand the service they need by giving them more knowledge. Women want choice, services which are genuinely geared towards their needs, and to take part in decision-making about their own treatment. This is not just a women's problem, for many working class men or black people face similar obstacles, yet it is important that women fight for specific demands because they have specific health care requirements. Only through working in groups can women hope to achieve any change, even though Women and Health Courses can be considered marginal to struggles within the health services. Nevertheless, it is important to continue to look for ways to influence these services and the providers of health care. Keeping long-term goals in mind is not always easy, as often the women and tutors felt powerless to change the immediate structures, but we argue that it remains important to maintain this broad perspective in the courses.

Progress within the WEA

Women and Health courses have had an important effect on the WEA in one particular district and we shall describe this example in order to show how mutual support and development can take place between women and health work and adult education provision in a wider sense.

The tutor/organiser for Women's Studies in the North West District was contacted by a local group campaigning for a Well Women Clinic. The group wished to develop some form of educational provision alongside their campaign, and together we decided to hold a day school on Women and Health in June 1982 to which over 50 women came. At the end of that day, when we asked whether there would be any support for a follow-up course, the response was practically unanimous. Armed with this information, we contacted the local branch of the WEA and asked if they could include such a course in their autumn programme. The branch committee decided against this, despite the overwhelming evidence that the course would have no recruitment problems. After some consultation with the District Secretary, the district decided to sponsor the course directly. The local branch complained about this because they felt that it raised issues of local democracy and branch autonomy, but the district felt that it could not ignore such an obvious request from so many people in the area. The course went ahead, attracting well over 60 students to many of the meetings – perhaps rather a large number for satisfactory teaching purposes, but showing the great demand for courses. Much of the course was collectively taught by members of the Well Women Clinic group, who also did the bulk of the work normally done by active branch members, organising publicity, booking the room and collecting fees.

Subsequent events have shown that this experience convinced members of the group of the relevance of the WEA and the role it could play, not only in the area of Women and Health, but over a range of topics. This first course has so far led to the establishment of five others in surrounding areas, all of which are being organised by local women. Early in 1983 some of these women met other women, and men, from the area to discuss the setting up of a new WEA branch in Stalybridge – an area hitherto without a branch – and this branch has now been established. Although coming from the stimulus of Women and Health courses, the branch programme is a broad one and this shows how new students brought into the WEA through Women's Studies Courses can strengthen the whole organisation.

We have now reached a stage where, in order to maintain and increase development of this work, more resources will be necessary. Many, although not all, courses are free and the provision of child-care at classes also means that the cost of each class to the WEA is greater than usual. Yet, instead of seeing such factors as a barrier to further developments, the attitude at district level is encouraging, and the WEA is aware of the value to the organisation of continuing to make progress.

The most important step forward has been a successful application to the Health Education Council in 1984 to extend women and health work within the North West District of the WEA. This new project aims to reach a wide range of women of all ages in the Greater Manchester area and, in particular, working-class women and those who are economically disadvantaged, including women from ethnic minorities. The project started in April 1984 with the appointment of two full-time workers who were to build up networks of contacts and initiate new courses, and it is to run for three years and involves teaching, developing materials, training, dissemination and research. Women within the networks that are to be established, and those on the courses, all have a voice in the content and direction of the project and in this way the workers hope to initiate the growth of a movement which will last beyond the life-span of the project itself.

Apart from the local focus, the project workers intend to develop a resource pack and activity kit which can be used for other courses elsewhere in the country. The pack will include guidance for those who wish to start a self-help group and practical information on how to run a group. There are other efforts to reach those women who do not attend courses, including an idea to produce a newspaper-format publication on women's health for wide national distribution to health centres, GPs, clinics, Community Health Councils, and so on. The paper would contain practical information on a range of women's health issues together with suggestions on how readers can become involved in courses and campaigns. Finally, the project will be evaluated by a research programme and the results will be disseminated in order to gain wide publicity.

For both the WEA and the HEC this project is an exciting development which opens up new areas of investigation and work. Different ways of reaching women and of organising and giving support are to be explored, and the commitment to develop the skills of local women to act as tutors of self-help groups is an important step forward in strengthening local networks. As we are both involved in this project we hope to report on its progress in the future and point towards the way forward.

Conclusion

Obviously no single course can solve all of women's health problems, and no course exists independently of the wider social factors which conspire to keep women in a position of subordination. But we do feel that, through their involvement in Women and Health courses, many women have begun a process whereby their experiences and knowledge are validated and their strength is encouraged. For different women the courses have provided different ways forward; for some we hope they have gained greater personal confidence and better physical and mental health. Others have become involved in the women's health network in the area, become volunteers in well women clinics and even tutors on other health courses.

In spite of our clear enthusiasm for Women and Health courses we realise that we cannot avoid addressing two questions: what can we realistically cover and achieve in one course? and where do we go from here? The first question will partially provide the answer for the second. In one course we can perhaps cover a wide range of topics but the depth of coverage and the extent to which the course can promote change depend on factors not always within our control. For example, if the course is attended by women who are personally dynamic and active in local initiatives it is easier to build on their desire for collective action. On the other hand, if the course is attended by women who mainly want to learn in the more traditional way the outcome will be different.

A final consideration is the extent to which we can see a course through to its logical conclusion if we are not of the local community. Perhaps the Stalybridge example shows us the way forward because it demonstrates that, with support from WEA tutors, a group of women can generate sufficient energy to organise a course and the necessary follow-up activities. Women and health courses can then provide skills, impetus and new ideas on which local groups can draw to develop their future activities.

References

Birke L & Gardner K (1982) *Why Suffer? Periods and their Problems.* London: Virago

Doyal L (1983) Women, health and the sexual division of labour: a case study of the women's health movement in Britain. *Critical Social Policy,* **3** (1), 21–33

Evans M (1982) In praise of theory. *Feminist Review,* No 10

Graham H (1984) *Women, Health and the Family.* Brighton: Wheatsheaf Books

Laws S (1983) The sexual politics of pre-menstrual tension. *Women's Studies International Forum,* **6** (1), 19–31

Leeson J & Gray J (1978) *Women and Medicine.* London: Tavistock

McRobbie A (1982) The politics of feminist research; between talk, text and action. *Feminist Review,* No. 12, 46–59

Oakley A (1980) *Women Confined. Towards a Sociology of Childbirth.* Oxford: Martin Robertson

Phillips A & Rakusen J (1979) *Our Bodies, Ourselves.* Harmondsworth: Penguin

Roberts H (1981) *Women, Health and Reproduction.* London: Routledge & Kegan Paul

TUBE (1981) *Annual Report.* Manchester: Worker's Educational Association, North-West District, Manchester

Unemployment and Health Study Group (1983) *Unemployment, Health and Social Policy.* Nuffield Centre for Health Services Studies. University of Leeds

Workers' Educational Association (1982) *Classes with Childcare.* Workers' Educational Association Guide. London: WEA

3

A Feminist Perspective in Midwifery

MAVIS KIRKHAM

About the Author

I am 40 and I have been a midwife for 14 years. I live in Sheffield, and I have two daughters and have lost a baby.

I left school at 15, and then held various jobs, travelled, and sporadically acquired a varied education, but it was through politics that I came to feminism. Workers' control has been my important political concern, and I have seen something of this in Jugoslavia in the early 1960s, in producer co-operatives in various settings, and in the first ujamaa villages in Tanzania. Only much later did the growth of the women's movement enable me to make the crucial link between the need for control in one's work and the same needs throughout my life in my own body.

Because of this background, and the fact that I work with women's bodies, I am very aware of the points at which these needs produce stark contradictions, and of the power relationships that haunt these contradictions.

I originally did my nursing training to gain a useful skill to take back to Tanzania, but then I did midwifery training and found the energy around birth so powerful that I have stayed in this field every since.

I have written this chapter very much from my own experience as a hospital midwife who has had the opportunity to do some research on midwifery care during labour. This research was made possible by a DHSS Nursing Research Fellowship. I am now responsible for antenatal teaching and my work is based in a hospital antenatal clinic, but I also work regularly on the labour ward. I am very aware that what I have written leaves out vast areas of midwifery, especially the work of community midwives.

AIMS

The word 'midwife' seems to me to mean in concrete terms exactly what 'feminist' means ideologically: with woman. I want the

35

women I care for to have confidence and faith in their own bodies, and really to 'tune in' to their selves and their children. They need to take responsibility from the start for the great responsibility of parenthood. Our society does not help women to trust their bodies, so as feminist midwives we need to offer a setting where women can learn a great deal and feel confident to make choices, knowing that we will support them.

A midwife brings her technical skills to care for a mother and her baby, but the essence of these skills is the very quiet art of ensuring that the woman is safe and strong. Often the important thing is not to act, but to be there to ensure that the woman feels safe to do what she feels is best. Perhaps the difference between being the ring-master and being the safety net is really the difference between doctors and midwives.

Woes of the hospital midwife

Midwifery is defined as care during and around normal birth. The midwife is with the woman at crucial points in pregnancy, and throughout labour. She helps the woman to give birth and she supports her later as she gains confidence and strength to care for her baby and resume her life.

Midwifery has a long and proud but largely unwritten history, although much was written to malign midwives by the rising male doctors who saw them as a great threat (Donnison 1977). Today, I feel that a crucial part of a feminist midwife's work is the defence of normality in the face of male-dominated obstetrics and its attendant technology and medical ideology.

Women still have a right to choose the place of birth of their children, and if we lose that right many other choices in childbirth will be lost too. Feminist midwives inevitably work to maintain that right in reality, and to support women in their choices. I find I do this mainly through women's groups outside my actual job.

The vast majority of births in this country now take place in hospital, and I work in a hospital. Hospitals are strongly hierarchical institutions and in such a setting the place of women, whether as staff or patients, is usually at the bottom. The underlying values which led to the centralisation of maternity care in hospitals largely dictate their structure, and therefore give rise to the problems of women within that structure. Hospitals exist to centralise medical expertise (largely male) and equipment (expensive and largely male-designed) for maximum efficiency, and women come (at whatever cost) to the experts (often in order to be told to rest). The woman is the consultant's 'patient' and he controls the 'care' of 'his' patient, although he may never see her. Such a hierarchy of institutional expertise limits the autonomy of its workers as well as those it serves.

Midwives still cherish their description as practitioners in their own right but as normal birth moved into hospital the reality behind the definitions changed. Previously all pregnancies were seen as normal until judged otherwise, a judgement usually made initially by the midwife. The reverse is now true, as all pregnancies now fall under medical management and are 'normal only in retrospect'. By this logic, the midwife as practitioner in her own right is defined out of existence. The hospital midwife's work therefore becomes either obstetric nursing or what medical staff define as provisionally normal and are therefore prepared to delegate. Fortunately, in practice, it also embraces the vast areas of work which doctors either do not have the time for or do not see as important. Doctors are expensive and in a hurry but pregnancy and labour are long, as is the real work of the midwife.

Nursing and midwifery, too, have strongly hierarchical power structures. The way the nurse or midwife feels her position within this structure greatly affects those she cares for. As Sheahan (1972) observed of American nursing, 'If power corrupts, so much more so does powerlessness. It corrupts by changing our perceptions of ourselves ... being too subordinate, too alienated or too weak to effect change.' Our training within hospitals and our socialisation as women make it all too easy to accept the constraints imposed upon us. Yet by our example we teach the pregnant women to accept them too. We are the ones who spend time with the women, and it is our actions which teach patients to be patient and to accept the system. We do not have to do this. We know it is not healthy.

We who are with the women can listen to them and encourage them to listen first to their own bodies and their babies. There is immense scope to do what we believe to be healthy within the National Health Service despite its structure and, ironically, the present cuts give us more scope whilst giving us much more work.

We are there to care for those women and therefore we must work to improve the system, but never in a way that will hurt the women it serves. I feel that confrontation between midwives and doctors usually falls into this potentially hurtful category. I have often seen a confrontation between doctor and midwife acted out, sometimes years later, on the body of a woman who was not part of the original confrontation. This poses terrible dilemmas, but together we must be able to find wiser ways of moving towards real change. Through our own research and teaching we can alter attitudes, and a wide range of political channels are open to us as women and as midwives.

There is also a contradiction between much-needed fundamental change and the ways a feminist midwife can make the best use of our present, inadequate system. I have chosen to concentrate in this chapter mainly on the details of everyday life as a midwife, because this constitutes my working life and because I believe that change will come through struggling at this level. The maternity service certainly needs to be transformed – but it also has to exist. So we find ourselves, with assorted companions, fighting the dismemberment of the old monster which is the NHS while at the same time seeking to change it from within.

PRACTICE

Antenatal care

It seems to me basic that all antenatal care should be of immediate use to the pregnant woman. A great deal is learnt at antenatal clinic and these checks should be a source of information for the woman herself and not just for her file. We can make it a basic rule to do nothing to the woman without her agreeing to it, and understanding why it is done and what is learnt from it. There is little point in weighing a woman without telling her the result in terms she understands and how much she has altered since her last weighing. This leads on to talk about nutrition, fetal growth and body image – which is what antenatal care is for. If we record her weight and do not tell her, our silence says 'this does not concern you' and across such a void she will not voice her concerns.

Pregnant women really want to learn about their bodies and every test gives us the opportunity to help them. A low haemoglobin can be dealt with from the starting point of 'What do you like to eat that's got lots of iron in?' This takes longer than an order to 'double your iron tablets' or 'eat lots of liver' but achieves better results. She might even feel brave enough to mention that the tablets give her constipation, and therefore piles, or that she loathes liver.

Surely there is no excuse for ever taking a woman's blood pressure without immediately explaining what we hear to the woman, even if the doctor is waiting? Sometimes I still find this difficult if the doctor is impatient, but if we do not do it our example teaches the woman that saving the doctor's time is more important than her understanding.

In some places women now check their own urine with help. Pregnancy is about discovery and taking responsibility, and these principles should apply to all we do.

Palpation is the centre of antenatal checks: it is our opportunity to feel the size and position of the baby and, while giving a running commentary, help the mother to feel the baby as well. From this she can understand her discomforts caused by pressure from the feet or head of a lively baby. We can listen to the fetal heart and she can, too, if we use technology appropriately. Later in pregnancy she can hear the baby directly with a stethoscope and an 'X' can mark the spot for her partner to listen at home. We can explain what we hear as women explain what they feel. This is what antenatal care is for, and it must not be sacrificed however long the queue for the 'conveyor belt'. Otherwise there is no point in the waiting of those in the queue.

We owe this not only to pregnant women but also to student midwives. In some places midwives are not trusted to give antenatal care, but I feel that only if we demonstrate that we can give good care – and that it takes time (something doctors do not have) – will we be entrusted with it.

Pregnancy is also an opportunity for more formal teaching. This is the midwife's field and it is a large one. Antenatal classes are an opportunity for women to gain knowledge, confidence and courage, yet many antenatal classes consist of a midwife in uniform lecturing rows of silent women. We all remember from school how such a system did more to teach us our place than to realise our potential, and this kind of layout says to a woman as she enters the room 'be quiet and listen to the expert/midwife'. Yet as midwives we have suffered so much from 'experts': how can they know these women's needs?

This rigid approach to antenatal teaching by midwives may spring from feeling nervous and ill-prepared and therefore hiding behind our routine and uniform, for we are well-trained to insulate ourselves from patients when we feel insecure. Women are perceptive, and if we hide like this they will collude with us and will not ask questions which may challenge our stance as experts. Thus we create a charade which helps no-one. Only when we can see women as allies in a wider search for knowledge and change, and can accept the limitations of our own training, can we really help them to learn. Only if we help women to learn about the things that worry them will they feel the basic confidence neces- sary to make choices. I am asked lots of things I do not know, but if we find out together we are all better equipped for the future.

Learning is richer for all of us if it is shared sitting in a circle with pregnant women, mothers and babies without the barrier of uniforms. We cannot then control what is said, but together we can explore the contradictions and differing advice which they will inevitably meet. Some of the pregnant ones will then return with babies to enrich our future classes and to say 'what it's really like'. So together we help women to make the best of the system and of their experiences.

Labour

I see the midwife as the supporter and sometimes therefore the defender of the woman she cares for in labour, but to achieve this we must really concentrate on the woman and her needs. So often there is a contradiction between expectations that the midwife will be in control of her working situation (and the doctor of his) and the mother's need to experience labour according to her own preferences. We face so many more contradictions in other staff's attitudes to us if 'our' patient is noisy; our hope that she may stop swearing in transition as the senior nursing officer's round approaches; our feeling as the woman turns to us and says 'What do you really think?' while the doctor stands in the doorway; our arthritic knees when she chooses to squat for delivery; our frustrated desire for experience of alternative birth positions when she opts for an epidural anaesthetic ... And how often is pain relief given to the mother to relieve the discomfort of the midwife?

We need support for ourselves, but we also need to spell out our dilemmas so that we can face them as such, rather than just as 'midwives' distress' manifest as a retreat once again behind our uniform and procedures. We need to share skills, and there is much we need to learn if we are not to lose our nerve and encourage that passivity in patients which gives us greater control of our working situation. There is great skill in knowing when a woman's progress in labour can be best helped by an intravenous drip, a walk, suggesting that her husband should take a walk, a deep bath, a shoulder massage, or a good laugh. These skills are not learnt during our training; we learn them by taking responsibility for our own education, but in doing so we risk the ridicule of those we work with.

Women on a labour ward can learn what to do or what to expect by taking their cues from us. If we give information they will feel free to ask for more, but if we deflect or ignore their questions they will not ask again. In my research with midwives and patients, I heard exchanges like these:

Patient: How long does it take?
Midwife: Babies come when they're ready. (changes subject)

Patient: I like to know what is happening.
Midwife: You'll be an expert soon. (silence)

Patient: I don't know what to expect.
Midwife: You don't with your first. (end of conversation)

None of these women asked another question during their labour, though there was a lot they wanted to know. Student midwives learn these techniques for blocking or deflecting the woman's search for information from the midwives with whom they work. The woman in labour learns appropriate behaviour from those who care for her, and if we prefer her to be passive she probably will be. What an indictment of us!

In labour, as in pregnancy, there is no place for empty reassurance like the following example from my research:

Patient: I'm scared.
Midwife: You mustn't be scared. (silence, delivered 8 minutes later)

By saying 'You mustn't be scared' or 'Don't worry' the midwife implies 'Shut up', and the woman's ensuing silence shows she receives this message. But the eight minutes of silent fear must have seemed eternity when a few loving words could have made them triumphant moments.

In my study of communication in labour I found many women adopting techniques such as self-denigration as ways of gaining information about the progress of labour from the midwife. Fat women were particularly skilled in this and repeatedly mocked their own bodies. Others used similar tactics of self-denigration in often referring to themselves as 'a baby' or 'a terrible coward', and the techniques worked. They did visibly put the midwife at ease and increase the flow of information, but what a sad situation they reveal among women.

Women in labour are very sensitive to the cues we give, as these examples show. But they also reveal how, by our actions, we can greatly increase their confidence in themselves and in us. In trying different ways of making a woman comfortable we state our priorities, and she will be free to tell us when she feels uncomfortable. If we tell her what is happening, she will feel free to tell us her worries. If we give a running commentary on our actions, we give information. If we say what we are about to do just before we do it, we give her the opportunity to say 'yes' or 'no' or to make choices without having an exhausting discussion. I have always felt grateful to the midwife who taught me this by her example.

As well as being aware of the cues we give out, we must be very aware of the cues a woman in labour gives to us. Does her fist pressed into her hip suggest back pain which may be helped by massage, movement or epidural anaesthesia? Does the tightly closed mouth show muscular tension inhibiting the opening of the cervix? If so, how can we best get her to smile? Do her repeated enquiries about her husband's comfort suggest that we need to help her to centre her mind more within her own body? Or does it suggest she is hoping he will leave? How should we respond?

I am sure that feminist care in labour is grounded in minute observation of the labouring woman's reactions, and not just in monitoring her pulse, blood pressure and fetal heart rate, and we can learn much about this from older, experienced midwives who may not call themselves feminists.

Many women we care for in labour will have different views and attitudes to ours, but we should always find the cues to what each one feels and wants. She may need to feel mentally in control and coping, in which case we must ensure that she copes in her own terms and is not trying to be a 'good patient'. She may need to sink deeply into her body as it takes over from her mind, and we are her guarantee of the privacy essential for such regression. She may feel overwhelmed; sometimes 'for patient's information' is the best reason for a vaginal examination though it is not one of the official indications. She may just be scared and only we can help her leave the labour ward as brave as a woman needs to be with her new baby.

It is easy with an articulate woman who has a well-worded list of her requirements in her hospital notes (and feminist earrings to cheer our hearts!). Although she will have ideological battles with 'authority', she is of the social class for which the system was built. The working class woman, the black woman and the woman who does not speak English want care and information just as much, but their realistic assessment of the situation tells them they are unlikely to get it. So we need to be very sensitive to their cues, although we may face many dilemmas in trying to provide them with the feeling of safety which every creature needs in labour. Perhaps being a feminist on a labour ward means learning Urdu at night-school (as well as counselling, yoga and biochemistry!).

We have to cope with men on labour wards as doctors and as partners. Both suffer tiredness and stress, which most men are not accustomed to coping with sensitively. To be 'with woman' we often stand between her and the man, which is not an easy place to keep a foothold. We inevitably compromise to keep going, but we can try to monitor our own responses and actions.

There are tensions between being 'with woman' and 'with doctor', even though we are all working to help the woman. If attending to the doctor means that we are neglecting the woman's immediate needs, should we ask for help? We may fear that this will be seen as our inability to cope, so we 'cope' by neglecting the woman just when her discomfort is likely to be greatest, and in doing so we state our priorities.

There are many ways we can help her partner or friend to support a woman in labour, although often we need to be very unobtrusive so as not to inhibit the experience between them. We can teach him massage, we can use his knowledge of the ways she expresses tension to help him ensure that she stays relaxed, we can explain, and we can often gently move his attention from the machinery towards the woman and her needs. Often it is useful to show him how to behave so that it is less likely that he will be asked to leave should abnormalities occur. Occasionally, we take the role of authority when she feels she cannot cope with his presence, but does not want to live with the consequences of saying so.

Not all labours are as women hope they will be. In inductions, 'caesarians' and all abnormal situations, women's need to understand what is happening and why becomes greater, and they need support so that they can cope with the experience in the way that suits them best. Although midwives are basically concerned with normal labours, we are just as much present and needed with the abnormal. Here the doctor's skills are central and we experience the contradictions between the nurse's role, seen as doctor's aid, and the midwife's role 'with woman'.

Not all experiences of labour are good or fruitful, and here too we take our cues from the woman. She must feel safe enough to express her loss, her pain and her disappointment, and we may express our emotions to the point where they help her feel safe. Beyond that we need to know where to find support for ourselves, elsewhere.

We need to build on our labour wards a framework within which we can give and receive support and counselling in sadness, mourning and disappointment. Once there is a framework within which we, as midwives, can really talk, then perhaps we could use it to learn, too, from each others' good experiences. How do we build such a safe framework within the existing power structure?

Language in labour

We are very much at the mercy of the language of our society – its words, its concepts and the values behind them – and this is particularly true for women on a labour ward. The language of the labour ward is the language of obstetrics which measures the objective progress, or otherwise, of a labour, and such measurements are often not given to the woman. There are no words in that language to describe the woman's perceptions of labour or the care she feels she needs. In expressing, or simply experiencing, the labour subjectively she is therefore likely to feel at odds with her attendants, whom she seeks to please. When this is so, she apologises.

In my research study most of the women I observed in labour apologised. Many apologised frequently if they felt they were not behaving well, were 'being a nuisance' or 'causing trouble' by making requests or simply receiving routine care from busy staff. The commonest words I heard women say immediately after delivery were 'I'm sorry', usually addressed to the midwife. Clearly the habit of apology comes from life outside the labour ward. Nevertheless, to use it there the woman must accept an external standard of behaviour, which is that of the staff, against which she judges herself to be inadequate. Most of those staff are midwives! We may not control our work setting, and it is not our language either, but we accept the apologies which acknowledge the power structure!

In the strategies used to gain or give information without 'causing trouble' to the basic order of the ward, there are striking parallels between the actions of mothers and midwives. These tactics are not unique to labour but are developed over a lifetime, or career, of coping from an inferior position. Patient apologises to midwife, junior midwife apologises to sister, sister apologises to doctor. Similarly, each observes and learns by indirect means rather than asking questions and thus confessing 'ignorance' and risking discomfort. Midwives, as much as patients, lack an appropriate language and in adopting the language of obstetrics they adopt too its values and its limitations. Yet it is these very limitations which ensure the continuation of midwifery.

We need to build a language *of* women *with* women in childbirth, and women have been working at this for a long time. Concepts such as 'transition' are very useful for women and necessary to antenatal teaching, though they are not seen in obstetrics textbooks. Yet because midwives' training is in the language of obstetrics, these concepts of language and of caring are not developed and handed on. Only if we raise our voices will the beginnings of our language be heard, and only if we share experience can we build concepts which are of use to women.

If we share our skills they will be handed on, and we must also describe them for those who cannot stand with us and watch. True midwifery research is much needed in this area.

Postnatal care

Postnatal care is very much the midwife's field. It seems logical that most of this care should take place at home and the woman should start as early as she wishes to live with her baby in her own setting, with all necessary support and help provided. The community midwife knows the reality of each woman's home situation and should be able to ensure all necessary support, from home helps to family rallying round and breastfeeding counsellors. But in reality community midwives are so often very thin on the ground, the few home helps work only with the elderly, and women having first babies are expected to stay in an alien and unrestful hospital for about a week. Here, as in all midwifery care, we need to work to change the system as well as to make the best of the existing situation.

Midwifery care of the new mother should be centred on helping her to take responsibility for her baby and get as much rest as possible. Many women need a lot of help in the early days of breast-feeding, and shortage of staff at this stage can be very damaging. New mothers and babies need time and care from the midwife when *they* need it, yet so often the solitary midwife on a postnatal ward has to complete the 'essentials' (form-filling and the statutory daily examination of mother and baby) and has no time to care. Postnatal midwifery does not appeal to those orientated to the care of passive patients because it is about taking responsibility and discovering self-reliance. New babies and mothers are notoriously impatient and unappreciative of hospital routines, and perhaps this is why this area is so starved of human resources.

When most harassed, hospital staff tend to fall back on rigidly enforcing the rules. Should we be encouraging first time mothers to leave hospital sooner so that family and friends can rally round? Or would this simply overburden the domiciliary midwives? Should we be checking that the ward is 'ready for visitors', or encouraging families to come in and really help? So often accepting help from outside is seen as an acknowledgement of failure, or a threat to our shaky professional status. But should we be preventing others from doing what our service cannot do? Breast-feeding counsellors, for example, or Muslim families bearing appropriate curries can only improve postnatal care. But experienced breastfeeding mothers may not echo the hospital policy, or the curries arrive at the appointed meal times. Can we take these risks with the order of the ward?

New mothers have a lot to learn. They need to be able to trust their carers and to rest, and here a midwife is like a mother. If the woman knows she can ask for help and that the midwife will make herself available and listen then trust grows, but women will not 'trouble' us if we are 'busy'. If, for instance, the tired mother says she wants to breastfeed then she can only rest if she can trust the midwife not to impose her own views by bottle-feeding her baby while she is asleep.

Coping with the abnormal is an even greater challenge, yet somehow tired newly-delivered women can find the strength to help those suffering if we trust them. I once worked on a ward where four women and babies shared a room, and at first three of the women showed unease and envy that the fourth received more attention from the staff, and her husband was allowed to visit for much of the day. I remember very apprehensively getting those three women together and telling them that the fourth woman's baby could only live for a few weeks but, after sitting and crying, they went back to the room and they really loved that woman and her baby. They cared for her as I never could with the rest of the ward to care for: they shared her anxiety, anger and mourning and she accepted them and their normal babies. I admired them and they made me braver as a midwife.

Mothers have a phenomenal capacity to rally round and this is especially true if they have similar experiences. An important part of a feminist midwife's job, therefore, is knowing how to link those who have had a particular experience by putting them in touch with the women's health network and the many specialist support groups. Linking women with others makes them stronger, and I find it very satisfying to introduce a new mother to one who has survived postnatal depression, breastfed a baby with a cleft palate, or speaks Spanish, for example. The domiciliary midwife has great scope in this way to help women out of their isolation once they have returned home.

SUPPORT

So where does the feminist midwife get her own support? She certainly needs it and probably does not get it from her immediate superiors, and I would have given up years ago without the Association of Radical Midwives. ARM started in 1976 and its aims for the benefit of childbearing women are to

1   re-establish the confidence of the midwife in her own skills;
2   share ideas, skills and information;
3   encourage midwives in their support of a woman's active participation in childbirth;
4   reaffirm the need for midwives to provide continuity of care;
5   explore alternative patterns of care; and
6   encourage evaluation of developments in our field.

ARM national meetings enable us to get together and talk about the things we need to talk about. By discussing the problems and contradictions in our work we each feel less isolated, and by learning about other midwives' practices, feelings and skills we are able to improve the care we give and bring about change where we work. We share skills, our knowledge grows, and together our language develops, and these meetings also give me a real transfusion of hope and enthusiasm.

We now have ARM regional groups which meet regularly, and it means a lot to me that there are other midwives in ARM who I meet in the hospital where I work, because this gives us support and the opportunity to talk about our practice with women who share our values.

ARM is an essential support group, but few of us work every day with other feminist midwives. I think a feminist midwife gets her everyday support from other women, and this may be from consciousness-raising groups, feminist health groups or other women's organisations. Consumer groups involved with maternity services offer much mutual support on a local and national level. The National Childbirth Trust, Association for the Improvement of Maternity Services, and several other groups share many of our aims, and a great deal has certainly been achieved in my local area through working together. These groups also provide essential information on what is happening elsewhere, and knowledge of precedents can help us to improve the services we give and not repeat mistakes made in other places.

Above all else, the women we care for will also care for us if we trust them. This goes against our training, which implies that the patient is not trustworthy, but only if we trust the women we care for will they feel able to trust themselves. It is this personal trust which I, as a feminist, feel is essential for women and especially for mothers. If we trust and support them, they will also trust and support us.

As a feminist midwife I do not seek to confront the system, but to help women to beat their own paths around and through that system. The satisfaction of being a midwife comes from constantly stretching, just a little, what women feel they are able to do. It is a circle, for I am convinced that change in the maternity services can only come in response to pressure from women themselves. If I help them to feel braver in getting what they want from the maternity services, then they will ensure that the role of the midwife will remain vital and cease dissolving into that of obstetrician's handmaiden.

Acknowledgements

I would like to thank the midwives from ARM for their support and many useful comments on this chapter.

Useful Addresses

Association for the Improvement of Maternity Services: 19 Allerton Grange
  Crescent, Chapel Allerton, Leeds LS17 6LN
Association of Radical Midwives: Lakefield, 8A The Drive, Wimbledon,
  London SW 19
National Childbirth Trust: 9 Queensborough Terrace, London, W2
Society for the Support of Home Confinements: c/o Margaret Whyte, 17
  Laburnum Avenue, Durham

References

Association of Radical Midwives (1982) *The Practising Midwife: 2nd Annual Conference Report.* London

Donnison J (1977) *Midwives and Medical Men: A History of Inter-Professional Rivalries and Women's Rights.* London: Heinemann

Gaskin I M (1977) *Spiritual Midwifery.* Summertown, USA: The Book Publishing Co

Kirkham M (1983) Labouring in the dark: limitations on the giving of information to enable patients to orientate themselves to the likely events and timescale of labour. In Wilson-Barnett J ed. *Nursing Research.* Chichester: Wiley

Inch S (1982) *Birthrights.* London: Hutchinson

Sheahan D (1972) The game of the name: nurse professional and nurse technician. *Nursing Outlook*, **20** (7), 440–444

4

A Feminist Perspective in District Nursing

MARY TWOMEY

About the Author

I was one of those people who always wanted to be a nurse, although I was often discouraged from considering nursing by teachers and family friends who regarded nursing as low status work. When I left school I was fortunate in securing a place at university to do a nursing degree, combining academic work with practical nursing and so pleasing everyone. My subsequent feelings about nursing have swung from enthusiasm to disillusion, despair and eventually a firm commitment to working for change.

I found nursing to be much different from what I had expected. Particularly hard to cope with was the rigid hierarchy in hospitals, which seemed to militate against caring. I also disliked the exaggerated respect given to doctors and the unreasonable demands they often made of nurses. My growing feminism encouraged me to be assertive in situations I found distressing, much to the dismay of some of my tutors. I was regarded by a few as a 'difficult' student.

Much of my support at this time came from friends who were involved in the Manchester Politics of Health Group and then from the Radical Nurses Group. This helped to focus my ideas and also gave me the strength to go back into the situations which were the source of my dissatisfactions. No amount of encouragement, however, could help me to survive midwifery training and it was after abandoning this that I took up my present job as a district nurse.

My work as a nurse is to some extent complemented by my involvement in the women's health movement. This includes teaching sessions on Women and Health courses, helping in a Well Women Clinic, and involvement in a local women's health group. My own health is also very important to me and for me being healthy means feeling fit, which I achieve by playing squash regularly and by walking and climbing. So health and health care is a dominant theme in my life, from a personal perspective through to a political perspective.

District nursing tends to be regarded as the poor relation of hospital nursing – a low technology alternative for those of us who can no longer cope with the pace of the modern hospital and are content to potter along with the same group of patients year in, year out. Stereotypes of district nurses persist, helped along by the occasional appearance in a television serial. We continue to be seen as rather motherly women who are not too clear about our facts but who nevertheless have our hearts in the right place (Twomey 1983). Whilst I personally do not feel particularly motherly, I have rejected the high technology pace of the hospital, not because I cannot cope, but because I became increasingly frustrated by the lack of opportunity to use my caring skills within an institution whose priorities seemed to be set largely around medical interventions and where I spent most of my time ministering to the needs of the hospital and the doctors, rather than to those of the patients.

All district nurses, with the exception of some nursing auxiliaries, have come through the hospital system: some of us training as State Registered Nurses and some as State Enrolled Nurses. Although I worked as a staff nurse on a hospital ward for only a few months after qualifying, most district nurses have worked as enrolled nurses, staff nurses and ward sisters on various wards for several years before choosing to come 'on the district'. This is not a choice which is made lightly as district nurses now have to undertake statutory training, with some nurses taking a drop in salary before qualifying.

District nursing, as Monica Baly points out, is not hospital nursing in a different setting, although many of our patients are referred to us by the hospital, for example, after surgery or after 'rehabilitation' following a stroke (Baly 1981). Although we care for people of any age who require nursing, the majority of our patients are elderly, many of them being elderly women. The health problems of the elderly are not ones which can always be quickly solved, therefore care may be needed for several months or years. Such care demands a different approach from the often short-term nature of hospital care and the limits on relationships between nurses and patients that this imposes. Developing long-term relationships with patients requires additional skills to the technical ones emphasised in hospital training, and demands a respect for the elderly which is not often found in the present health care system. Developing these relationships based on respect is for me an essential part of my work.

Relationships with other workers

Just as most district nurses have received their basic training in the hospital setting, so have the GPs with whom we work. Thus GPs perceptions of community nurses are influenced by their experiences of or relationships between doctors and nurses in hospitals, where the dominance of the medical profession is largely preserved (Salvage 1985). So, many GPs still see themselves as controlling or directing the work of district nurses and as delegating tasks to them (Dingwall 1978). This is contrary to the concept taught on most district nursing courses of a primary health care team consisting of social workers, community nurses and GPs who make equal contributions to patient care and should be awarded equal status.

Establishing equal working relationships depends on all those involved being willing to communicate with each other about their different roles and ideas. This communication has not been widely developed, however, and the situation in Britain mirrors that described by Jo Ann Ashley in the USA:

> 'Medicine has passed down tasks to nursing practice as medical care has become more developed and technical, but physicians have not been willing to communicate with nurses to learn their views about who does what in health care and why.'
>
> (Ashley 1976)

Since 1974 district nurses have become 'group attached' in many areas, which means a particular group of nurses working with the patients of a particular GP practice, rather than working on a geographical basis. It was hoped that this would develop a team approach, so facilitating better patient care, although nurses continue to be employed independently of GPs. Developing good communications is clearly difficult if one member of the team sees himself as superior to or more important than the others. This inequality is not just reflected in who is seen as having ultimate control over what happens to the patients, but also in social relations within the 'team'. So whilst the GPs always call me by my first name – Mary – I continue to refer to them as Doctor X or Doctor Y. I feel that the nature of relationships between GPs and community nurses also reflects the fact that many GPs are men, whilst nursing remains a predominantly female profession. To quote Ashley again:

> 'Physicians seldom perceive nurses as anything other than the women with whom they work, and nurses relate to physicians not only as a nurse to a physician, but as a female to a male.'

It is interesting to me that it is since I have started working with three women GPs that I have become more acutely aware of the different ways in which we address each other – I am used to talking to other women as an equal! Previously I had worked with three male GPs where the problems were even more acute. I have been told by one GP, for example, that he would not talk to me before I smiled! I cannot imagine this being said to a man! On another occasion I was harangued for ten minutes on the phone by a GP for having made a nursing decision without consulting him first. Again, I could not imagine this happening to a man. As Christine Webb points out, we have a double hurdle to overcome as women and as nurses if we want to establish ourselves as an independent caring profession (Webb 1983).

Working with other nurses

The nurses who work with each group of GPs are themselves organised into district nursing teams, with the number of nurses depending on the size of the practice. Until very recently I worked with a team of three nurses with myself as the district nursing sister being the co-ordinator of the team, whose other members were a nursing auxiliary and a State Enrolled Nurse. As this shows, the hierarchy within hospital nursing still exists in the community setting, although it is perhaps adhered to less rigidly. This caused great problems for me when I first started working as a district nursing sister. As a feminist I am committed to breaking down hierarchies and yet as a nursing sister I am in a position of power and am also responsible for the care that is given to 'my' patients. I am also paid considerably more than the auxiliary with whom I work and so cannot expect her to take equal responsibility for care. My initial solution to this problem was to ensure that I did as much of the 'caring' work as the other nurses so that I would not be thought to be using my status to offload the heavy physical work, but also to complete the referrals and assessments, and keep records up-to-date, whilst making sure we all met daily to discuss our work and share ideas. This situation has eased somewhat as I now work with a much smaller caseload and only one other nurse, but I still feel involved in a juggling act between my ideals and the reality of my work situation.

Working closely with other nurses has also meant that I have had to confront issues which are central to my feminism. I strongly believe that women should not be expected automatically to take on the care of sick and elderly relatives for example, but this is a view not shared by all my colleagues – women are still expected to be very involved in caring. This is an issue which tends to be discussed in relation to individual situations, but it is often useful to broaden it and ask whether we, as independent working women, would be prepared to take on the role we expect so often of others. Using personal experience works well here – my response to nurses' criticisms regarding infrequent visiting by daughters or sons is to talk about my own infrequent visiting of my parents, because of the particular tensions that exist in my family. I sometimes wonder, however, whether I am criticised as the 'absentee daughter' by the district nurses who occasionally visit my parents!

The issues of racism and antisemitism within nursing are probably the ones that I find most difficult to confront with the nurses with whom I work. White nurses, for example, continue to assert that black people have a very low pain threshold, and criticise elderly Asian patients for not being able to speak much English. Confronting racist attitudes is something which I continue to struggle with and which involves dealing with my own racist assumptions as well. I know, for example, that I tend to assume that patients referred to me will be white, rather than not making any assumptions about their colour. When relating information to each other, other nurses will always mention that a patient is black. This is something that I avoid but it is not a strategy that works well, as another nurse will always add the missing information. Obviously we still regard white as 'normal'. I feel I also need to develop a more effective strategy towards antisemitism, because antisemitic remarks by nurses are very frequent. As a feminist I feel personally committed to confronting antisemitism and racism but this is not something which can be done solely on an individual level – nursing as a whole needs to develop effective anti-racist strategies.

Relationships with patients

One of the most distressing aspects of nursing and medicine that I encountered during my training was the lack of control which the majority of patients had over their care. Despite the increasing popularity of the concept of the nurse as the patient's advocate, I frequently felt powerless when faced with situations where patient's needs were being ignored. It was this feeling of being a powerless observer in the face of some extremely distressing incidents which contributed to my decision to abandon midwifery training and take up district nursing, where I felt that more equal relationships could be established and it would be possible to hand back some control to patients.

Of course, control cannot simply be handed back without any changes in the system which generates the inequality. Simply by deciding to try and establish more equal relationships with patients I am exercising some control, and I very much control the nature of relationships that are built up with most patients. With a very few of my patients I have developed important friendships and have been able to receive as well as give support, but with the majority it is still I who decide how involved to become. I also find it virtually impossible in the present system to give patients full control over their care. I remember when I started district nursing being sure that I would not coerce patients into going into hospital against their better judgement, but I soon found myself desperately persuading people to be admitted in order to give their relatives a much needed break.

Trying to support both patients and relatives can also lead to conflict – whose needs do you consider first? It is very easy to exclude either relative or patient from the decision-making, or to focus on the needs of one whilst ignoring the other. I find this particularly difficult when I am involved in situations where a man is caring for his wife or mother. Women are expected to, and do, care for relatives much more than men and many women have a lifetime of caring (Walker 1983). Recognising this means that when I am working with women looking after a male relative I am keen to ensure that their needs are thought about as well, although having your needs thought about is a far cry from having them met. Because of the way we regard women as natural carers, it is often accepted by both patients and carers as normal for them to take on this role. When a man is looking after his wife or mother, however, the situation becomes more confusing, with the carer less able to cope and the patient often distressed with less acceptable roles – it is more acceptable for a woman to bath a man than vice versa, for example. I feel that women in these situations do tend to get less good care from their relatives than a man would, and they are often very distressed at being so dependent. However, it is also impossible not to feel a great deal of sympathy for men trying to care for their female relatives and finding it very unfamiliar and frustrating. Trying to support both carer and cared for in this situation can leave one feeling torn in two opposite directions. Support cannot be unconditional, either – I have occasionally worked with male carers who have been abusive and threatening towards me, situations which create conflict between my understanding of their frustration and my anger as a woman being physically threatened by a man.

People need more than support if they are to have a say in the kind of care and treatment they receive. They also need information about what is happening to them and what alternatives are available. Wanting to give patients more say in their treatment can sometimes lead to a conflict of interests, however. I have often felt very frustrated at having to abandon what I believe to be the most appropriate treatment for leg ulcers, for example, because the patient has no faith in it. In such situations I have often caught myself saying 'I know it hurts, but. . .'. In other words 'I know best'. Conversely, it can be equally frustrating when, having presented someone with various options, they prefer me to make the decision, saying 'You know best', although it may be unfair to ask people to make decisions about confusing treatments, particularly when they have never been expected to have an opinion about their treatment in the past.

Working with women patients

The women's health movement has provided much anecdotal evidence of the poor quality of health care received by women, particularly in obstetrics and gynaecology (Doyal 1979). Again, women have little control over the treatment they receive, and very often do not know what has been done to them. On several occasions I have visited women who have had a hysterectomy and found that they did not know whether or not they had had their ovaries removed as well – a vital piece of information for most women. The fact that these women do not know whether they have had their ovaries removed reflects their lack of involvement in decision-making about their bodies. Sometimes women are very unhappy about having had such surgery, feeling they would not have chosen such a major operation if they had been fully consulted.

Visits to people who have had surgery and need stitches removed or wounds dressed tend to be short-term and not a major part of our work. Often, however, I find myself returning to see women to talk through and explain what has actually been done to them and what the implications will be. This frequently involves explaining basic anatomy and physiology, which should have been done before surgery. Giving women information after surgery seems like shutting the stable door after the horse has bolted – had they had it prior to surgery, they might feel more confident about their treatment, as well as having that opportunity to question and consider it. However, belated though it may be, I still feel this information is essential. The problem is that it is also time consuming – explanations about how your body works cannot be given in five or ten minutes, but spending longer means less time for the rest of the morning's work. Unfortunately, the counselling aspect of district nurses' work is not widely recognised, and it is often difficult to justify to others why you have spent an hour simply talking to a patient who is not seriously ill.

Spending time talking to women about their illnesses and treatment can also involve helping them to look at different approaches to their treatment – helping them to take control. This can often be very difficult for them to do when faced with the supposedly superior knowledge of the medical profession, especially as patients are usually seen alone by doctors, and any suggestions from a nurse might be seen as out of place. Encouraging patients to take more control and look at their illnesses more holistically can work, though. A woman I had been visiting for nearly two years refused her third lot of surgery for a postoperative infection, knowing that I would continue to visit and support her. Together we looked at changing her diet and trying some herbal remedies. Amazingly her infection cleared and the wound healed within weeks. Another patient of mine was unhappy about being given high doses of steroids following an ileostomy and we looked at ways of reducing stress in her life, as well as developing strategies to cope with the doctors who wanted to maintain high steroid levels and think about future surgery. Working with women in these situations often makes me despair at the narrow focus of medicine and makes me excited about the potential scope of nursing.

This narrow focus is also reflected in the treatment women receive for stress and anxiety. In my previous practice many women used to come to my weekly clinic for cytamen (Vitamin B_{12}) injections after having been to their GP complaining of tiredness or lack of energy. Often their symptoms were a result of their home circumstances or an emotional upset such as a bereavement, which no amount of added vitamins would help. Whilst there was little I could do myself to help such women, I frequently encouraged them to go to one of the local well women clinics, where at least they would have a chance to talk about their situations in individual or group settings and try to gain support and explore alternative solutions.

Only a few women, however, will actually go to a well women clinic – many more will continue with their monthly cytamen injections and their tranquillisers. Working with women in this situation can be very depressing, knowing that I do not have the time that they need and very often knowing I have no solutions to offer. Many women feel particularly depressed and vulnerable following the death of their husbands, and need long-term support. Although we do continue to visit people after a patient we have been looking after has died, we cannot provide the depth of support needed, partly because of lack of time and partly because we have not been taught the necessary skills. Voluntary organisations such as Cruse help some, but there are many more women who are not getting much-needed support.

Through my work as a district nurse I became aware of the inadequacy of the health services offered to women on the housing estates where I worked. Although I could only deal with problems on an individual level, it was obvious that more than this was needed and together with a friend I helped to organise a women and health group which is campaigning for better health services for women in the area. Participating in this group allows me to challenge what is offered by the health service more effectively than if I were simply working from within it.

Working with elderly women

A very large proportion of my time at work is spent with elderly people, particularly women and men over the age of seventy-five. Many of the problems we help to overcome arise from increasingly limited mobility, perhaps as a result of arthritis, strokes or conditions such as Parkinson's disease. But as well as dealing with the physical consequences of immobility, such as incontinence, we are also very involved with the emotional consequences which can include intense loneliness, loss of self-respect, and despair. It is perhaps working with these problems that is the biggest challenge to us as district nurses, and to do so effectively I feel that it is important to look at our own views and prejudices towards elderly people and particularly towards elderly women.

Just as many of our patients are elderly, the majority of these patients tend to be women, and often single women whose husbands have died many years before. A survey conducted by Hunt in 1978 found that 29 per cent of women aged 75–84 live alone, with 44 per cent of these having done so for more than twenty years. When infirm, elderly women do still live with their husbands, they are likely to receive help from district nurses and home helps, as men are not expected to be able to look after elderly, infirm relatives (Land in Walker, 1983). To some extent this explains why we care for more elderly women than men. Elderly men are often cared for by their spouse or by their daughters, and these women receive little help. Chris Phillipson wrote that

> 'large numbers of men retire in a poor state of health and it is often forgotten that the burden for their care will almost inevitably fall on the wife.'

Whilst women outnumber men in the sixty-plus age group by 50 per cent, among those over seventy-five they comprise nearly 70 per cent of the total, and it is predominantly women who face old age as a period of loss and abandonment (Phillipson 1982).

It is this sense of loss and abandonment, together with physical disabilities or chronic illness, that gives rise to the despair and depression I often encounter in the elderly women I visit. I have very frequently heard patients wonder why they are still alive and maintain that they look forward to death as a release from a meaningless existence. Inactivity accompanies depression, and suggestions of visits to day centres or visits from 'good neighbours' are frequently rejected. I can remember long conversations with one woman in particular, at the end of which we concluded that the problem was largely mine in that I found it very difficult to accept her lack of enthusiasm for life. Rather than helping her by suggesting various 'activities', I was pushing her to accept services that she definitely did not want, probably so that I could feel that I had done something.

Pushing elderly people to accept interventions they do not want is something that I feel happens frequently in community care. We all have our ideas about what is best for people – 'she should not be here' or 'she would be happier in a home' is commonly said. I sometimes find it difficult to hold on to my belief that it is the elderly person who should decide what is best for her, and that most people prefer to stay in their own homes if they are given adequate support. Too often decisions about going into residential care are taken without considering the feelings of the person involved, and district nurses may collude in this. After all we have easier access to social workers, GPs and geriatricians than most of our patients do.

Part of the reason for excluding elderly people from decisions about their future care is probably due to a belief that they do not have valid opinions. This lack of respect for elderly people is reflected in the way we treat them and talk to them. I continue to find it extremely distressing when nurses assume that 'elderly' equals 'deaf', and automatically shout at people. However, I am not immune from these stereotypes and it is even more embarrassing when I find that I am shouting too! Not shouting, however, is not enough. Because of the negative images elderly women receive of themselves, it is important to assert your belief in their right to make decisions on their own behalf and actively to seek their opinions on various issues. One patient I visit infrequently was amazed when I said: 'People think that when you are old you have no opinions'. She had recently decided not to go into an old people's home despite worsening arthritis, and was obviously finding it difficult to justify her decision. I also think it is important to remember that elderly people have a past – a wealth of experience which we can draw upon to inform our current practice. I have often been encouraged by elderly women patients when talking of my wish to remain independent and unmarried. Most of our patients have made the same decisions as we are making – whether to marry or not, to have more children or not, to change jobs. Also, as Gladys Elder pointed out,

> 'to understand the old it is essential to have some idea of the social, economic and educational factors that have moulded them.' (Elder 1977)

If we are working so closely with elderly women, I feel it is important to counter the popular stereotypes of elderly people as passive and weak. This means confronting our own prejudices, and prejudices which persist in nursing. It is not unusual to hear a nurse describe a male patient as 'like an old woman'. What does this say about the expectations we have of elderly women patients? It seems to me impossible to encourage their self-respect if we ourselves have no respect for them. Also, what does it say about our feelings about ourselves? After all, we will be old women one day. I feel that many of these questions are central to feminism as well as to nurses. Phillipson points out that in Britain feminists have largely neglected to consider the position of elderly women – much of what has been written has dealt with the problems or needs of those caring for the elderly. If we are to confront stereotypes we need to start listening to elderly people themselves.

Carers

Being attentive to the needs of carers is also vitally important.

Many of the carers we work with are women – a survey of carers carried out by the Equal Opportunities Commission (EOC) showed that there were three times as many women carers as men. As Walker points out, when politicians talk of community care, 'community' and 'family' are euphemisms for 'female relatives' (Walker 1983). As cuts in health service budgets increase, so dependency on relatives for care increases, and it is becoming harder to find even short-term relief for carers. This situation often presents me with the dilemmas of wanting to avoid asking female relatives to take on the bulk of caring work, but at the same time being forced to rely on women to carry out the majority of the care, because we do not have the resources to do otherwise. We are now in the situation where help which was being given is being withdrawn from some women, so increasing their work. A less obvious way of denying care is to accept the status quo – it is very easy to visit a patient for the first time who has been looked after for several years by her daughter, for example, and to assume that this will continue, without asking the daughter if she needs relief from such physically and emotionally exhausting work. As someone who strongly believes that women should not be expected to take on the primary care of relatives, I experience a lot of conflict in working with women carers to whom I am able to offer so little help. As a district nurse I might arrange visits once, twice or even three times a day, but these visits will rarely last even as long as twenty minutes or half an hour, leaving the carers to cope for the remainder of the twenty four hours.

Given that carers are providing the majority of the care needed, they will have a good understanding of their relative's needs and the best way to approach many of the problems that might be encountered. However, this expertise developed through experience is not always recognised by district nurses, and it is very easy to 'take over' control of the care someone is receiving. As nurses it is important to us to believe that we have skills and knowledge which equip us to provide good care. It can be difficult to accept that a carer might actually have more skills than us in dealing with a particular patient or situation, perhaps because we feel relegated to the role of helper. But, if we are expecting relatives to continue to give care, we must also be prepared to let them have control over the situation in which that care is carried out. One way in which we deny carers a measure of control is by not stating a definite time for visits, on the basis that we do not know how long each visit will take. I feel sure that, with a little time and thought, we could give most patients an approximate visiting time, which would then allow carers and patients to plan their day. We all know how frustrating it can be waiting in for the plumber or the gasman – imagine being in this situation every single day! Just as providing patients with more information can help give them a chance to participate in decision-making, so we can give carers more information too. It is very easy to by-pass relatives and relay information directly to social workers or GPs, for example, who might then visit unexpectedly or make further decisions. Other health workers exclude relatives also. I have often arrived at someone's house without them knowing I had been asked to call. I feel that if we are going to continue to ask relatives to take a large part in caring, we need to recognise that it is probably they who are central and we are peripheral to that care in many cases. As a feminist, I also believe it is important to campaign for increased resources for the elderly and chronically sick so that women do not have the burden of caring forced upon them.

Lack of resources can make supporting women carers difficult not simply from a physical point of view but also from an emotional point of view. Often the needs of the carer are very different from the needs of the patients and it can be difficult to support both. Looking after someone who is frequently incontinent, or who is bedfast but constantly in need of attention, can be very frustrating and many women express feelings of anger towards these relatives. This anger is easily understood, but women often need a great deal of support and encouragement not to feel guilty about feeling angry. It is also easy to understand the fear and discomfort of patients who need so much attention, and of course they need support as well. Conflict arises when it is clear that the carer needs a break but the patient is very unhappy about going into hospital for a couple of weeks. Often the carer experiences this conflict as well, recognising her overwhelming need for rest but at the same time feeling guilty about seeing her relative distressed. I remember one patient in particular whose daughter was often extremely depressed and exhausted by her care, but who found it very difficult to let her mother spend two weeks in hospital. Unfortunately, this lady died whilst away, which compounded her daughter's feelings of guilt.

Being a source of support for carers can sometimes mean more than giving physical and emotional support. Just as we are encouraged to think of ourselves as the patient's advocate, so we must also be prepared to act as the carer's advocate too. I have attempted to do this on several occasions and it has often been very difficult and painful. On one occasion I had repeatedly to telephone hospital consultants and registrars and argue that a patient desperately needed to be admitted to hospital. This man was seriously ill and very aggressive, and his wife found it impossible to cope with him. On this occasion I was lucky in that I had the support of a community psychiatric nurse who could also see that the situation was untenable. Eventually, the patient was admitted to hospital but we were horrified to learn that his discharge was planned for a few days later. In this case I visited the hospital ward and wrote in the patient's medical notes that neither the district nurses nor the patient's wife were in a position to accept responsibility for his care were he to be discharged. In fact, the patient died the next day. Unfortunately, such situations are not rare, but it takes a considerable amount of courage to argue with doctors who control admission to and discharge from hospital beds, and who have a limited number of beds to go round. Although doctors do not control nurses' actions they still have a great deal of power and influence which can be difficult to confront on an individual level.

Maintaining a feminist approach

One of the problems I find in working as a district nurse and being a feminist is that I sometimes feel quite isolated at work. I do not know many other district nurses who are feminists and those that I do know live scattered around the country, so opportunities for discussion about my work are fairly limited. Much of my approach to my work has been built up through experience which has either developed, changed or modified my first feelings about the job.

Whilst I still believe that it is important for women to be given space to talk of how they feel about being ill and the treatment they are receiving, fears about the future and their problems at home, I also feel it is important to let them define the extent of the relationship that develops between us. It is important not to push women into discussing their fears and problems, particularly if I can only offer them a little time in which to do so. Perhaps this is one of the most difficult things to accept – that women might want to talk, but not necessarily to you. Or they may not want to talk at all.

When women do want to talk about what is happening to them, then, for me, being a feminist means being prepared to listen, to encourage and to explain. Listening and encouraging can be straightforward, but explaining can sometimes be a lot more difficult. I think it is important to acknowledge when I do not know the answers to someone's questions, but it is equally important to be committed to finding the answers, if possible. This can mean telephoning consultants or their secretaries for information and knowing how to share this information if it is not good news. Being prepared to share knowledge and information can also be difficult in certain circumstances. Following gynaecological surgery, for instance, most women want to know what implications the surgery will have regarding their sexuality. This can be a difficult area to discuss, as many women feel embarrassed when talking about sex. Sometimes it can be embarrassing or uncomfortable for the nurse as well. I remember sitting on the settee with one woman, drawing detailed diagrams of the anatomy of the female reproductive system, and explaining the nature and effect of the surgery she had had, whilst her husband was sitting on one of the chairs opposite. Clearly she felt quite comfortable, but I did not.

Having established caring and supportive relationships with women it can then become very difficult to end those relationships when they are no longer in need of care. I think this is a problem widely experienced by district nurses, who continue to visit patients after their nursing needs have been met. In many cases it could be that, although their physical needs have been met, they still have emotional needs which require continued support but referral to other agencies seems inappropriate. Occasionally, however, it is simply difficult to say that you will not be visiting any longer. One of the hardest situations for me was leaving a woman I had been visiting daily for almost two years whose wound suddenly healed very quickly. It was not the regular dressing that this woman most appreciated, but the strength and confidence she felt she had gained through having constant support from other women who listened to and encouraged her. It seemed almost incidental that these women were district nurses who ostensibly came to dress her wound. Very often the difficulties of leaving can be avoided by promising to continue to 'call-in', but in my experience this never works because time is so limited and such promises are unfulfilled. If the way we establish relationships with our patients is important, then so is the way we close these relationships so that we do not leave people feeling bereft or abandoned.

It is often difficult to distinguish what is a feminist approach to district nursing from what is 'good nursing'. Although I would always identify myself as a feminist, my overriding identity, at least when I am at work, is as a nurse and I am probably more likely to think 'how should I as a nurse respond to this problem?'

rather than 'how should I as a feminist respond?' Being a feminist, however, has forced me to question many of the assumptions of nurses involving women's roles as carers and hierarchies within the system. Other problems which perhaps I notice more as a feminist include dealing with the sexism of male patients and relatives. In hospitals many nurses profess to enjoy nursing men rather than women. Personally I have never enjoyed nursing men and still find it difficult, although we have fewer male patients. Whilst I am personally relieved that we have fewer male patients, I am also aware that this is because they are being nursed by their female relatives – a situation which I firmly believe should be remedied.

One of my priorities as a district nurse is giving patients control over the care they receive. I started district nursing committed to this principle and remain committed to it, but I now know that it cannot be achieved without changes in the health care system within which I work. I cannot give my patients full control over their care but I can give them more information and be ready to respond to their needs or demands as flexibly as possible. I can also be prepared to act as their 'advocate' even when this is personally painful or difficult for me. I also recognise that there are some occasions when I will keep control – perhaps in situations where I feel personally threatened or where unreasonable demands are being made of me.

Just as I feel that some of my initial ideas about approaches to district nursing have been changed and informed by my experiences as a district nurse, so my work has informed my feminism. For me it is a dynamic relationship. The things I do as a feminist, such as being involved in well women centres and women and health groups, make me think about the way I work with women in the NHS. Similarly, the people and situations I encounter at work inform my feminism. Working with and considering the needs of elderly women make me aware of how little space the women's movement and the women's health movement have given to them. At times I despair of both feminism and nursing and I often feel I get little support from feminists over my dilemmas in nursing. But I am very glad that when, three years after starting my present job as a district nurse, people ask me how I like it, I can still reply 'I love it', despite its frequent frustrations!

Acknowledgements

Without the support of many friends I would not have stayed in nursing and so would not have written this chapter. Of these, I am particularly grateful to Anna Garry, Judith Emanuel, May Lubien-ski, Maggie Fortnam and Judith Gillen. I would also like to thank Sandra Sherlock and Margaret Tomlinson who worked with me when I first started district nursing and helped me to untangle my confused ideas. Thanks must also go to Bernadette Newton who typed the draft.

References

Ashley J A (1976) *Hospitals, Paternalism and the Role of the Nurse*. New York: Teachers' College Press

Baly M (1981) *A New Approach to District Nursing*, London: Heinemann

Brent C H C (1981) *Black People and the Health Service*. London: Brent CHC

Dingwall R (1978) In Dingwall R & McIntosh J ed *Readings in the Sociology of Nursing*. Edinburgh: Churchill Livingstone

Doyal L (1979) *The Political Economy of Health*. London: Pluto Press

Elder G (1977) *The Alienated: Growing Old Today*. London: Writers' and Readers' Publishing Cooperative

Equal Opportunities Commission (1980) *The Experience of Caring for Elderly and Handicapped Dependants: a Survey Report*. Manchester: EOC

Hunt A (1978) *The Elderly at Home*. OPCS. London: HMSO

Phillipson C (1982) *Capitalism and the Construction of Old Age*. London: Macmillan

Salvage J (1985) Nursing – behind the painted smile. *Spare Rib*, No 153, April

Twomey M (1983) The demands of district nursing. *Nursing Times*, 25 May

Walker A (1983) Care for elderly people. In Finch J & Groves D *A Labour of Love: Women, Work and Caring*: London: Routledge & Kegan Paul

Webb C (1983) Words fail me. *Nursing Times*, 6 July

5

Feminism and Health Visiting

JEAN ORR

About the Author

I became a feminist largely because of what I experienced as a health visitor working in a very personal way with women. This work coincided in the early 1970s with my discovery of feminist literature, and my reading provided a framework for understanding and guiding my practice. It seemed to me that feminism was particularly relevant to health visiting – a service largely provided by women for women. Feminist analysis helped me to place women's health within the wider context of society and helped to explain the tremendous discontent which women have with their lives, and which Betty Friedan calls 'the problem which has no name'.

I am now a lecturer in nursing at the University of Manchester and I have been involved in the well women's movement in the north-west of England, helping to set up well women clinics. At present I work with women's health groups and I am editing a book on women's health in the community. My interest is in developing a feminist approach to health visiting and working towards greater participation by women in community health initiatives.

Health visitors have identified four principles which are the bases of practice (see Figure 5.1) but as yet there has been little discussion of their implications for practice (CETHV 1977). These principles are political in nature in that they make explicit certain assumptions and beliefs underpinning health visiting. This is the case if we apply them to the population as a whole, but how much more political and controversial they become if we use them explicitly as feminists in our work with women.

Doing this would lead us to focus on women at the expense of men and would state openly our belief that women suffer from structural inequalities in society based on gender as well as class.

How might the application of these principles require us to see our concerns about women's health? It would mean recognising

69

Principles	*Examples*
The search for health needs.	Identify women who are thought to be 'at risk' and/or who are not receiving health services (eg. women who are battered or who are stressed by caring for dependent relatives).
Stimulation of the awareness of health needs.	Encourage women to campaign for a change in services or the development of a new service such as a Well Women's Clinic
The influence on policies affecting health.	Form a pressure group to increase the provision of cervical screening.
The facilitation of health-enhancing activities	Provide information to help women remain healthy (eg. teaching relaxation techniques or organising assertiveness training courses).

Fig. 5.1. Principles of health visiting (CETHV 1977)

the reality of the lives of women in political terms of access to scarce resources, and suggesting social and economic solutions to what are often seen as individual problems. Implicit in this is the concept of positive discrimination in favour of women. After all, if we choose to help run a Well Women's Clinic we are in practice withholding resources from other client groups.

Many health visitors may be disturbed by the implications of this stance and yet, as workers paid by the state, we play a political role in implementing Government policy. To support and implement the status quo is a political position, and we continually have to balance the needs of various client groups. Every health visitor is aware of pressure to become involved with a range of health-related activities covering all ages.

I am not suggesting that a feminist perspective is easy to implement with clients or to come to terms with at a personal level. It requires us to question whether we are forcing our own commitment to feminism on to other women who may not share our views and/or who – recognising their position – have made a conscious choice to support the status quo. What right do we have to encourage women to raise their consciousness if we cannot follow through with the help they may need? Are we to be just a different form of tyranny forcing women to confront aspects of their lives which are too painful for them to change? These are questions we still have to debate.

What is not in question is the relationship of feminism to health visiting and its effect on the outcome of health visiting intervention. Thorpe (1979) asks whether 'the role of the health visitor is to raise the consciousness of women, and in so doing, to challenge the role of women in society as a whole?'. This would, of course, involve the health visitor in challenging her own position as a woman, mother, or wife and, by definition, would lead her to challenge the position of health visiting itself in the traditional framework of doctor/nurse relationships. There is, however, a growing body of feminist literature which suggests that health care workers (including health visitors) are unsympathetic to the needs of women (Leeson & Gray 1978; Daly 1978).

We should be concerned about this lack of sympathy with a feminist perspective because of the influence that health visitors have upon their clients. Miers (1979), for example, says that health visitors are in the front line of care and prevention of depression and neurosis among married women. On a wider level in the community, the health visitor has been said by McKinley (1970) to be one of the most popular of the outside agencies. Caplan (1969) suggests that health visitors (as well as some other workers) may, because of their key position, be able to affect the mental health of families. While other social welfare agencies operate a crisis intervention service, the health visitor is the only worker who visits all homes with children and provides an outreach service.

That health visiting falls short of the expectations of feminists may not be all that surprising if we bear in mind the way in which health visitors see their profession in relation to society. Health visitors, as part of the wider social context, may enforce the values of a male-dominated society and their profession may reinforce these values because nursing (and health visiting) has a subservient relationship to the medical profession. I would argue that health visiting cannot be divorced from feminism for three reasons.

Firstly, the development of nursing and the status of women have been interdependent and often parallel (Glass & Brand 1975).

Other writers analyse the wider issues of the effect of the feminist movement on nursing. They tend to take what to many may be a radical stance, advocating the need for consciousness-raising groups in order to achieve personal and social change (Randolph *et al*. 1979). Kravetz & Sargent (1975) say that such groups attempt to develop both an analysis of society and appropriate politics based on the experience of being female. In doing this, the participants realise that the personal becomes the political. Bullough (1975) highlights the difficulties in the relationship between women and health care, and Colls (1980) suggests overcoming these by setting up a women's health care nurse practitioners' training programme where the emphasis is on education in areas of most immediate concern to women.

Shockley (1974) analyses the implications for nursing of a feminist perspective. She sees its change in the concept of femininity as having affected nursing practice in two ways. With different roles, clients bring different problems to the nurse counsellor and this change has resulted in some nurses rejecting the traditional nursing role in areas such as decision-making and self-concept. Bush and Kjervik (1979) examine nurses' self-image and suggest that nurses and women have not learned to value themselves and in consequence have not nurtured their own self image. The result of this could be that, if nurses and health visitors do not accept and value women, they will not seek to align themselves with the women's movement or place emphasis on the issues most relevant to female clients.

Secondly, feminists have analysed the ideological and value-laden role played by the state in family policy and health visitors should examine this analysis if they are to evaluate and influence policy. There can be few health visitors who are complacent about the current state of the family or the response of the Government to health needs in the community.

Even in the seemingly uncontroversial area of child development some feminists challenge the standard child development texts. Comer (1974) says that children in our society show a particular pattern of social responses because of the way mothers and children are isolated in the home. This social behaviour is then deemed 'normal' by the experts, which in turn encourages mothers in unsatisfactory and, indeed, harmful patterns. Comer maintains that the pattern of social development produced by this isolation reflects not the child's basic nature but the conditions in which the child is reared. Bernard (1974) shares this view and suggests that childrearing in many western countries compares unfavourably with methods found elsewhere. By assigning sole responsibility for child care to the mother and then isolating her from family and friends, demanding that she provide complete and continuous care, we harm both mothers and children.

Feminists who have analysed the family suggest that family relationships create and sustain the dependency and inferiority of women. Indeed, Leeson & Gray (1978) link husband-and-wife dependency with the inferiority of women. If nurses accept this role at home they are unlikely to be able to offer an alternative perspective to their clients.

Some feminists argue that, in order to upgrade the status of child care, men should be actively encouraged to participate fully in the care of children. Attempts to encourage fathers to attend parentcraft classes may be no more than token gestures, particularly when the content of many programmes remains geared to women. Simply to play about with words and call mothering 'parenting' will not break patterns of servicing in the mothering role unless men take responsibility for the personal maintenance of their own lives.

The institution of motherhood created by a patriarchal society ensures that women's potential remains under male control (Rich 1977). Dahl & Snare (1978) argue that the man acts as an agent of the state and enforces dependant patterns of behaviour on the wife and children.

Such a view of the family, as well as the myths and sentimentality woven by men about women as wives and mothers, creates conflict for many health visitors. Part of this conflict may arise because the feminist lobby has described the family in terms of oppression, and this is not what health visitors experience in their own lives, or at least it is not what they are prepared to admit.

Thirdly, and most importantly, there is a growing body of feminist literature relevant to health visiting. This literature identifies women's issues in relation to health care and may have implications for clients' expectations and the way they use health services.

Kjervik & Martinson (1979) bring together work which offers a nursing perspective for women in stress, and suggest that women in nursing should grasp, both personally and professionally, the health care issues confronting women. As women themselves, nurses have added insight into the stress and concerns facing a female patient. With their medical knowledge and self-awareness they can help ease the tensions facing women which are inherent in divorce, role expectations, battering, child abuse and the stress of loss.

Studies of women's needs have traditionally centred on mother-hood but now include issues which are much broader and affect many aspects of women's lives. Examples of feminist writings include work on coping with sexual identity crises after mastectomy (Kent 1975), the need for education in sexuality for nursing (Krizinofski 1973), the influence of feminism on psychiatry (Coppolillo 1975), problems of middle-aged women following family illness (Urban 1972), the effect of the women's movement on the occurrence of depression in women (Beck 1979), stress levels of divorced females (Tcheng-Laroche *et al.* 1979), and the grieving process of battered women (Weingourt 1979).

The relationship between health visiting and feminism will remain tenuous and uneasy unless health visitors make use of this increasing body of literature. Feminism has provided concepts about women's role and women's health which are crucial to health visitor education and practice and which help us to understand and analyse everyday situations. As a first step towards change, a feminist perspective needs to be critically examined during the Health Visitors' Course.

Health visitor education and training

As a teacher of health visiting, I am concerned about the sexism which exists in many institutes of higher and further education and is a continuation of what happens in primary and secondary education (Blackstone 1976). It is all the more serious, however, because in higher and further education, the assumptions are that the subject matter taught is somehow objective, value-free and scientific. This lulls students into believing that the perspectives of the social sciences are valid and all encompassing and must be 'correct'. According to Du Bois (1983), science is not value-free – it is made by scientists and is shaped by culture. Indeed, the closer the subject matter is to ourselves, the more we can expect our own beliefs to enter and shape our work. As higher and further education is an elitist and essentially male system of education (Evans 1983), we can argue that the theory generated within it is in fact grounded in and derived from the experience, perceptions and beliefs of men. To further compound this male theoretical view of the world, I would argue that these subjects are mainly taught by men, and men are in positions of power within the educational system. What female role models do students have, either within the health service or educational institution? Their experience is that men are in charge and that to succeed they have to please and placate them.

Existing courses for health visitors attempt to present the social and behavioural aspects missing from basic nurse training, but students tend to find it difficult to question and critically evaluate what is taught. In my experience, they tend to have difficulty at the beginning of the course in coming to terms with much of sociology and social policy's examination of class and poverty issues. This is mainly because students have middle class values and consider these subjects too 'radical'.

Students tend to accept the perspective presented on issues which most acutely affect them (eg. the analysis of the family and the role of women in child care). Furthermore, the social sciences do not fully describe the reality of their lives, their experiences as women being discounted and devalued. This is all the more worrying because student health visitors bring to the course a wealth of experience and observation of what it is to be female in our society. By the time they enter health visitor education, they have been intimately involved with women throughout the hospital system and they have nursed (and perhaps been nursed) in many settings. In my experience they fail to recognise the sexist nature of health care, and its effect on women patients and on themselves, and have no understanding of the political forces which operate in society to make women the victims of violence, poverty, low self-esteem, and illness.

A study of student health visitors' perceptions of women (Orr 1980) showed the extent to which they were influenced by sex-role stereotyping. Women were seen as passive, dependent, sentimental and afraid of change, with little control over many aspects of their lives. Women were said to have characteristics of warmth and expressiveness, while men were said to have characteristics in the competence realm. Women were also seen to suffer from little disadvantage in education, career, legal, financial or health care aspects of life. There was little awareness of the social divisions within society, let alone any awareness of the degree of sexual inequality.

Essentially, health visitor students have a patriarchal view of the world, and there is little evidence of any other perspective being presented during the course. What they receive is a male view of the world, masquerading as science.

Feminists have shown that there is no psychology of women, no sociology of women, no anthropology of women, no real history of women and no thorough and coherent social science theory about women. Bernard (1973) sees sociology as being that of the male world, and it was not until Oakley (1974) that we had an analysis of housework, although sociology has examined male work for many years. The problems and priorities of women were regarded as less important and main areas of childbirth and child-rearing have been ignored or only examined if they pose problems for the male world.

Much social science describes the male as normal and the woman as abnormal, deviant or problematic (Spender 1980), and women are continually described in relation to men (ie. mother, wife, lover). Westkott (1983) describes this as woman being cut off from her body and personal power, and being a person who mirrors and validates men. These perspectives were not questioned until recently and it is not difficult to see why.

Scientists did not listen to women or see our experiences as legitimate. Because men control language, we had no words to 'name' what we experience or feel. What positive words do we have to 'name' the rich and varied feelings of motherhood, birthing or menstruation? In terms of sexuality, women's experience is defined and named in relation to men. Brownmiller (1977) shows us the extent to which changing the language changes the power basis when she quotes Mehrihof as saying that if women were in charge of naming then the male-focused term 'penetration' could become the female-focused term 'enclosure'. What a change this makes in the balance of the relationship and sex-act!

It may be useful at this point to examine what Spender (1980) has highlighted about the 'inaudibility' of women in motherhood, as this has particular relevance to health visitors. According to Spender, motherhood in our society has a legitimated meaning which is equated with 'feminine fulfilment and which leaves women consumed and replete with joy'. While it is the case that motherhood can have this meaning for some women, Spender argues that it is only a partial meaning and it is false to portray this as the only meaning. Health visitors are aware that motherhood may have been a difficult and traumatic experience for many mothers but because these mothers cannot relate to the legitimised meaning of motherhood they are left feeling inadequate, estranged and isolated. There is no adequate space within the meaning of the word 'motherhood' to accommodate their experiences. If this is the case for the word 'motherhood', it is possible that the meanings of other words are also inadequate. The work of Oakley and other feminists raises questions for health visitors about how much they should be involved in helping women validate their experiences as opposed to helping perpetuate essentially male values and meanings.

Implications for health visiting practice

What can we do as feminists who are health visitors? We have the great strength that we are women working mainly with women and, as such, are in a key position to help women achieve their optimum level of health and wellness. We can do this, firstly, by working individually with women, secondly, by working collectively with women's groups throughout the community and, thirdly, by influencing colleagues and policy-makers within the NHS, local and central government, and voluntary organisations.

We can attempt to deal with the real concerns which women raise by listening to what they want and not imposing our definitions of reality on their lives. We can re-affirm with women that they have a responsibility and a right to look after their own health and we can offer them support and knowledge to facilitate this, even if it means a change in our practice and service provision.

Our practice should involve regular in-depth health assessment of the women we visit (Orr 1985 – see Figure 2). I know that many health visitors would maintain that this is too time-consuming, but the experience of my students who have undertaken it shows that it brings about a positive change in the relationship with the woman and focuses attention on the woman herself. I would also suggest that women would at least remember the visit and might understand a little more about the work of the health visitor. Such an assessment leads on to teaching women about things like stress reduction by relaxation or exercise, and involves the 'laying on of hands' for breast examination and, perhaps, demonstrating massage techniques for tension or headaches.

As feminists we have to develop a critical approach to our professional relationships with women and recognise that the model of the powerful professional is one which is antithetical to establishing positive rapport. The interaction should be one of equals, with the woman being seen as the expert on herself and her family.

One new programme which incorporates a different approach to clients and emphasises women's health is the Child Development

General Physical Health	Life Style	Social Activities and Relationships	Women's Wellness
1 Current state	1 Level of nutrition	1 Support systems	1 Menstruation
2 Current treatment	2 Weight	2 Sense of isolation	2 Pre-menstrual tension
3 Illness/accidents in last year	3 Smoking	3 Control over life	3 Menopause
4 Concerns with:	4 Drugs	4 Enjoyment of life	4 Vaginal health
(a) digestive system	5 Alcohol	5 Stressors and coping mechanisms	5 Cystitis
(b) bowels	6 Exercise		6 Breast examination
(c) skin	7 Rest/recreation	6 Depression	
(d) reproduction	8 Stress reduction		
(e) urinary	9 Work hazards		
(f) dental	10 Contraception		
(g) headaches	11 Sexual functioning		
(h) sleep	12 Reproduction		
(i) others			
5 Preventive screening			

Fig 5.2   Women's health assessment (Orr 1985). Reproduced by kind permission of Blackwell

Programme (Barker 1984), which is supported by the Bernard Van Leer Foundation of the Hague. It is a large-scale intervention study which involves health visitors and it focuses on altering the human environment surrounding the disadvantaged child during the earliest years of life. It is currently being implemented in five health authorities in England and one in Eire. There are five basic elements in the study:

1   It concentrates entirely on influencing the immediate environment of the child rather than working directly with the child.

2   Both the principal and secondary caretakers in the child's environment, the mothers and fathers, have been encouraged to seek their own solutions to the problems of childrear-

ing, with help and advice rather than take direction from health visitors.

3   The concepts and strategies used are simple, work-a-day, and intimately related to life among the disadvantaged.
4   Large-scale and rigorous monitoring has been undertaken to assess the quality of the reported achievement.
5   Changes have been made to the service pattern and functioning of the health visitors involved.

There are no set programmes or formal lists of behavioural goals for either parents or children. The health visitors have been trained to approach parents flexibility, discussing with them methods of stimulating the development of the children and how to overcome any development problems. The visit focuses on seven fields of development: language, social development, cognitive development, pre-schoool educational development, nutrition, health, and general development.

Each health visitor is given a large range of cartoon material with accompanying guides covering these areas. Between two and four cartoons are used as the principal focus of the visit, and the parents can study these in depth between visits. The health visitor completes a record of social and health conditions and also records the extent to which the mother (or father) has carried out the developmental tasks agreed at the previous visit. A new set of developmental tasks is discussed during the visit, with the mother (or father) being encouraged to put forward her (or his) own ideas for the coming months. The emphasis is on seeking solutions to problems which are both acceptable to the mother in her environment and developmentally useful.

This is a complex and wide-ranging programme and, at the risk of over-simplification, it may be useful to summarise its unique and important features:

1   It stresses the importance of working with parents and recognises that parents are the experts on their child and are in control.
2   A pattern of regular monthly visits is made, by appointment. The emphasis is on the health visitor sharing with the parents and eliciting a more in-depth response than may be possible in a traditional visit.
3   There is a recognition that, while the child is the focus, the health and self-esteem of the mother is also of crucial importance.

4   The health visitor herself does not put into practice ideas with the child, as this may make parents feel inadequate.

5   There is a positive approach towards the child's development and the parents are praised whenever possible.

6   There is an emphasis on the idea of childrearing being enjoyable – a concept which is often missing in other programmes which emphasise precise goals, tasks and achievements like some form of 'baby olympics'.

One aim of this programme is to raise maternal self-esteem and to give control back to women. As an example of this approach, the health visitor at the primary visit asks questions such as:

> 'Did you feel that, as a woman, you were in control of what happened to you during the birth of your baby?'
> 'Did the people who managed your baby's birth ask your opinion about how you wanted to have the birth – about position, injections, etc?'
> 'How much of what has happened to you in life is due to outside factors and how much to things within your control?'

Health visitors ask the woman what help can be given to make changes in behaviour, for example:

> 'Do you think it would be possible to cut down or stop smoking, at least for a while?'
> 'What help can I give you in this difficult task?'

While the main concern is with health, the woman is encouraged to explore other issues and offer solutions to problems, for example:

> 'Have there been any serious and unexpected worries or problems in your life over the past few years which might make it difficult for you to cope with bringing up your new child?'
> 'How serious were these problems?'
> 'Is there anything that you or I can do, or my colleagues, to help you overcome any problems that you may still have?'
> 'Thank you for being so helpful in answering these questions. It has shown what you and I can do to try to make things easier for you as a woman and a new mother'.

Feminism, then, offers us a different way of looking at health visiting practice and issues such as depression and violence against women. For example, powerlessness can be seen to lead to lassitude, self-negation, guilt and depression. Treatment for depression seen in the context of powerlessness is very different from prescribing tranquillisers and maintaining the status quo. Let us examine how feminism might help us to analyse three different aspects of our work: the family, violence against women, and primary health care teams.

Health visiting and the family

The whole notion of intervening in family life is a complex one and has within it tensions growing out of the relationship between the State and the family. On the one hand the family is seen as being private and personal, especiall when there are no children and the dominant values of society are being upheld. However, the State will often intervene when a woman becomes pregnant and will most definitely do so when the child is born. Reproduction is seen as a legitimate point of intervention, and pregnancy and childbirth result in the private family becoming the public property of professionals. After all, doctors decide and legitimise when a woman is pregnant and decide on the possibility of abortion if that is requested. The medical profession largely controls contraception, and social workers have a major role in deciding whether children should be taken into care. Health visitors make judgements about whether the parents measure up to professional expectations and the latest childrearing theories. To work with families is neither a value-free exercise nor is it easy for feminists, as the present emphasis in practice is mainly on reinforcing conformist types of behaviour and family patterns.

There are three models of intervention in family life which have differing underlying assumptions and outcomes, these are the child-centred, family-centred and professional-centred models.

The *child-centred model* has strong historical credence and institutional support in other areas of social policy. The proper focus of services is seen to be the well-being of the young child, with the needs of other family members being secondary. There is little recognition that there may be conflicts within the family, and help is only given if the safety of the child is threatened. In the case of the mother being abused, for example, help may depend on whether there is a risk to the child. Often, because of the strong focus on the child, other family health matters are seen to be marginal.

The *family-centred model*, while recognising the importance of children, tends to be more concerned with reducing stress and reinforcing family solidarity. The family is seen as a key social unit of society and its interests come before those of an individual member. Health visiting at present focuses its main attention on young children. While some health visitors may say that this is not the case, there is little evidence in students' family studies, for example, of any major emphasis on women's health. There may be passing reference to contraception or postnatal examinations, but students' work reflects what is taught and what is seen in practice and, therefore, reflects what I see as a major defect in current health visiting practice, which is a lack of awareness of the health needs of women.

A third model which seems to be emerging can be called the *professional-centred model*. This means that, as social and health policy changes towards community care, there is more involvement and control by professionals in family life.

The idea that families care for their needy, such as the handicapped and elderly, is not new (Rossiter & Wicks 1982). The new element is that the family unit and home are now seen as the desirable place for care, not necessarily because they are best but because the home will soon by the main, if not the only, place. Professionals must, therefore, use the home as a focus for their endeavour. This shift from ward to bedroom or living room raises questions about the role of professionals in controlling family resources and actions in the name of the State.

This model does not recognise any issues of conflict and there is little discussion of the issues surrounding the assessment of family need and little recognition of the value-laden nature of professional activity. There is little critical discussion about what it means to be a 'family visitor', and working with families is seen somehow to be a 'good thing'. Like the word 'community', the word 'family' is seldom used in a negative way. For example, we talk of being a family friend, restoring family values, maintaining the family unit and helping families to care for themselves. Within the professional domain, we talk of a 'good mother' as someone who has accepted her role and is willing to follow current childrearing theories. Implicit in this labelling exercise is the idea of 'normality', that is, a family which contains a husband, wife and children, despite the reality of family life in Britain in which this type of family is a distinct minority (Rimmer 1981).

Deviations from the so-called normal family are presented as problems needing special attention. Student health visitors appear to be encouraged to view the nuclear family as the norm and by implication, therefore, to measure all other groupings by this desirable standard. One-parent families, for example, are seen as deviant – even the label 'one-parent' depicts a degree of inadequacy: this is despite evidence that these families may be representative of an ethnic pattern of family life which is stable and well-accepted. Despite the emphasis on two parents, it is the woman's role in the family which is focused upon and prescribed and it is women who have contact with social and health services.

The State is largely concerned about the role of women as mothers and care-givers, and emphasises these roles to support the policy-shift to community care. It is not so concerned about the social costs imposed on women within the family (Rimmer 1983). Little interest is shown in women's health outside the medicalisation of childbearing and childrearing, and little concern with women who are seen to be deviant.

On health visitor courses, as we have seen, many of the subjects studied project a view of the family which reinforces women's traditional roles and also reinforces these aspects for the health visitor students in their own roles and their own lives and relationships. Dingwall (1977), in a study of health visitor education, found that students held an idealised view of marriage. Success for women was seen in terms of marriage and a family, not professional advance. Miers (1979) argues that much sociology, as well as the health visitor's training, idealises the family and indirectly seeks to uphold a sentimental or ideal model of family relationships, and Wilson (1977) shows how the State defines femininity, and how this definition is central to the welfare system. Woman is, above all, 'mother', and with this vocation go all the virtues of femininity. The female client is expected to wait patiently in queues at such places as baby clinics, to be ministered to either by a paternal authority figure such as a doctor or by a nurturant yet firm model of femininity provided by a health visitor or nurse.

Health visitors cannot reinforce these views of femininity and consider, at the same time, the possibility of change either for themselves or their clients. Increasingly, however, some health visitors are criticising the traditional perspective because it simply does not match the reality they face every day. It is within the family unit that we see children who are sexually abused and are the victims of incest. It is within families that women are battered emotionally, psychologically and physically. Living in a family can seriously damage your health yet there is a belief that any family is better than no family, irrespective of personal and social costs.

There is also an assumption that all members of a family benefit equally from membership and that the needs of each member can be reconciled with the overall benefits of the unit. Our life experience suggests that this is not necessarily true, but its implications for health visiting practice are seldom discussed.

The needs of the woman, man and child within a family unit are neither always consistent nor always incompatible, nor are they static. The family shifts in structure and function over time and in relation to circumstances. For example, the needs of a new family with young children clearly differ from those of a family with teenage children, and the relationship between the woman and man is different before and after the birth of a baby. It is difficult to ascertain whose needs are paramount within a family, to what extent conflict promotes survival of the unit, and to what extent health visiting intervention will be welcomed and utilised.

Violence against women

How does a feminist approach help us in our work with female victims of violence? Essentially it helps us to recognise that violence is a misuse of power and that its main victims are children, the elderly and women. It enables us to be aware of the possible extent of the problem (Binney *et al.* 1981) and therefore makes us recognise it as our legitimate concern. Health and welfare services are unresponsive to the needs of women in violent relationships (Borkowski *et al.* 1983) and indeed it was feminism which led the way in exposing violence and setting up a network of refuges.

As health visitors, our main task is to recognise the problem within our caseload. A study by Stark *et al.* (1979) showed that battered women had three times as many abortions and twice as many miscarriages as other women. Battered women were far more likely to be pregnant when injured, and kicking pregnant women in the abdomen has been described by other writers such as Evason (1982).

We should suspect abuse when we meet a women who has multiple injuries, when she is injured while pregnant or has a history of multiple or self-induced abortions, and when she reports persistent or vague medical complaints, has attempted suicide, has persistently used tranquillisers, or is anxious and depressed.

Women who have been abused make multiple visits to medical and psychiatric services for general health problems which superficially appear to be unrelated to abuse, but which are as much a part of the battering syndrome as the physical injury.

There are three suggested stages of battering. In the first stage are those women who have suffered repeated physical injury and minor medical or mental complaints. Those in the second stage present with physical injuries accompanied by more serious psychosocial problems, and so they are referred to psychiatrists. Women in the third stage have made multiple suicide attempts and present with severe medical or mental health problems. Abuse at this third stage often turns to self-abuse, and helpers see the symptoms as the cause of abuse rather than as the result. In other words, because the woman has severe mental health problems we can see why she might be battered. Many battered women at this stage are sent to psychiatric hospitals and day centres, where the approach is often to reinforce traditional female stereotypes. Putting on make-up and doing housework are seen as signs of recovery, and are the price to be paid for being 'cured'.

We must realise that much of our non-recognition of abuse is based on the model of care we deliver and the political biases we exhibit in defining need and allocating resources. The woman is seen as the problem *for* the family and not as a product *of* it. Battering should be part of the differential diagnosis we make, for the woman may be reluctant to state the problem overtly because of the stigma involved.

Health visitors and social workers may be the professionals most likely to discover victims and help them work out the nature of their needs (Borkowski *et al.* 1983). The general practitioner is often the key agent of first contact in the early stages of marital breakdown, but s/he may not see 'real' medicine as being concerned with marital problems. Borkowski *et al.* suggest that such problems should be referred to health visitors and that they should give victims clear information about legal and welfare entitlements, and advice on how to use other services and where to find emergency accommodation. There was concern that 69 per cent of health visitors interviewed in Borkowski's study said they had no knowledge of the law relating to battered women, and this lack of understanding of legal remedies may mean that clients are forced to take hard-line action which splits the family, when a cessation of violence is what they really seek.

We need to develop ways which will stop putting women in impossible situations concerning housing and money. We also need to address the question of client withdrawal from health visiting services, because this is often seen as an excuse for inaction by professionals. We become reluctant to interfere, even when asked, because of victims' real or apparent ambivalence towards the situation. On the one hand they still care for the man, but on the other they are afraid to stay with him.

Women seek help when in great distress but when the immediate crisis is over their priorities change, and fear of losing their home and possessions and breaking up the family force many back into the violent situation. This then makes helpers sceptical and reluctant to help again, but the value of such help, even if followed by client withdrawal, should not be underestimated.

There are two levels at which we can offer help. Firstly, at the individual level we need to consider battering as a possibility for women who present with medical and social problems. We need to accept the client's reality and not attempt to put our own interpretation on the 'facts'. We need to acknowledge the ambiguity of feelings, both our own and the client's, and be realistic about the scarcity of options open to her. Secondly, links should be made with women's refuges as part of the network of voluntary agencies in the community. It is essential not to fall into a 'blame the victim' trap, but instead to offer practical help and support, with due regard to legal remedies.

We should be aware in our work with families and in preparing young people for parenthood of the dangers of excessive disciplining of children and the perpetuation of sex-role stereotyping. We need to realise the sexism which exists within health and welfare services, and how professionals can reinforce the stereotypes of what is a 'good' mother and wife. Feminism helps us to recognise the extent of the problem and offers the means of intervention.

The primary health care team

The relationship between health visitors and general practitioners is a mirror image of the relationship between male and female in wider society. Indeed, health visitor students have been subjected to secondary socialisation in an occupation which epitomises the traditional position of women, firstly, as nurturant, passive and submissive mother-figure and, secondly, as handmaiden or help-mate of the male-dominated medical profession (Wilson 1977). The 'attachment' of health visitors to general practitioners is often discussed in terms of a 'marriage'. We can see, however, that once again health visitors as women are being described in relation to men as doctors. Attachment is an interesting word in this context, and if one asks health visitors to describe their work, they will often start by saying 'I am GP attached'. They are so used to being described in relation to men in private life that they automatically see themselves in the same way at work!

Health visitors and other nurses differ from doctors in terms of status, income and power and, while the rhetoric focuses on teamwork and sharing skills, the reality is that GPs are in control of their own premises and see themselves as head of the team. We are so used to men being 'head' of households, businesses, colleges, and so on, that we accept this without too much questioning. In addition, men take on the role as leader of a team because they are more familiar than women with the concept of being in charge of teams. They are socialised to be part of the pack, the scrum, the corporation or the regiment. Criticism of primary health care teams is often directed at health visitors, who are seen to have 'failed' to make a relationship and to explain their role to the doctors. They are expected to take on tasks such as immunisation to 'please the doctor'. In this case, health visitors carry out the procedure and doctors get paid. Is this another example of women economically supporting men whilst being seen as subservient to them?

Much of the literature which examines how the primary health team works can be likened to 'super-women' books because of its claim that health visitors would be more acceptable, more industrious, more accommodating, and so on, if they improved themselves. This emphasis on the performance of the health visitor and the extent to which she should change to facilitate the smooth running of the team seems to me to be an extension of the servicing function which women are expected to perform in the home. Why do we not ask doctors to change? Probably because we recognise that the 'good' health visitor does not confront or challenge the status quo of the male and the team. If she does challenge, she is labelled aggressive and unfeminine and denied access to the goodwill of the doctors and, in some instances, to the facilities and records.

Fortunately, not all health visitors subscribe to this model of teamwork but instead attempt to distance themselves from medical paternalism. This is not easy, as nursing managers and policy-makers dictate how and where health visitors function. It is possible to draw a parallel between the desire to keep health visitors within these teams, and so prescribe and control their work, and societal pressures to keep women under the control of men within the family.

We may be acquainted with issues of status and power between nurses and doctors from writings in sociology, and to some extent these are discussed during health visiting courses. What is not discussed, but is vital for any analysis of teamwork, is the sexist nature of language (Spender 1980). I suggest that Spender's book should be compulsory reading for heath visitors, to enable them to recognise how men control conversation by interrupting women in order to gain the floor for themselves and to prevent women from making points. The myth in our society is that women are the talkative sex, but research shows that it is in fact men who talk more in mixed sex groups, and who decree what is worth talking about and what is not. Therefore in any team meeting in which there is a mix of sexes (and this must be the vast majority), the nurses present, who are of lower status than the doctors (and in their own eyes are perhaps also lower in status than the social worker), are doubly disadvantaged. They are, without realising it, restricting their own opportunities to express their views by deferring to male interests and opinions. To deviate from this means being seen as dominant, bossy or aggressive. As Spender points out, 'when women are supposed to be quiet, a talkative woman is one who talks at all'.

If health visitors or nurses are to be effective in any team situation, these are the patterns of interaction of which they should be aware. For too long we have 'blamed' health visitors for the problems of teamwork, when the problem actually lies in the sexist and patriarchal nature of society. Until we acknowledge what is really going on within primary health care teams, we will continue to waste considerable energy and resources which could be better deployed.

Conclusion

A feminist perspective, therefore, has a major contribution to make in health visiting. It helps us to see the lives of women in feminist terms, and I suggest that all health visiting practitioners and students should read Rich's book *Of Woman Born* because it gives a vivid example of a feminist approach to motherhood. Rich presents us with two meanings of motherhood as the potential relationship of any woman both to her powers of reproduction (and to children) and to the institution of motherhood, which she sees as ensuring that that very potential – and all women – remains under male control. She presents a very different view of motherhood from that studied on health visitor courses, or indeed that recommended to potential mothers when she says, 'We need to imagine a world in which every woman is the presiding genius of her own body'.

I believe we can move some way towards that goal by using what has already been written about women's lives and women's health to guide our practice and health visitor education. A critical examination is needed of what happens on health visitor courses, and a recognition of the values and beliefs which underpin much existing education. Most urgently, we need to change relationships in health visiting by moving to a greater equality and by giving power and control to those we seek to help.

Of all the range of nurses working with women, I consider that health visitors are in a key position to effect changes in their lives. We have the means if we have the will.

References

Barker W (1984) *The Child Development Programme*. Bristol University

Beck C (1979) The occurrence of depression in women and the effect of the women's movement. *Journal of Psychiatric Nursing*, **17** (11), 14–16

Bernard J (1973) My four revolutions. An autobiographical history of the ASA. In Huber J ed *Changing Women in a Changing Society*. University of Chicago Press

Bernard J (1974) *The Future of Motherhood*. New York: Dial Press

Binney V, Harkell G & Nixon J (1981) *Leaving Violent Men*. London: Women's Aid Federation

Blackstone T (1976) The education of women. In Mitchell J & Oakley A ed *The Rights and Wrongs of Women*. Harmondsworth: Pelican

Borkowski M, Murch M & Walker V (1983) *Marital Violence: The Community Response*. London: Tavistock

Brownmiller S (1977) *Against Our Will: Men Women and Rape*. London: Penguin

Bullough B (1975) Barriers to the Nurse Practitioner Movement. *International Journal of Health Services*, **5** (2), 225–233

Bush M & Kjervik D (1979) The nurse's self-image. In Kjervik D & Martinson J eds *Women in Stress*. New York: Appleton-Century-Crofts

Caplan G (1969) *An Approach to Community Mental Health*. London: Tavistock

Colls J (1980) Preparing women: health care nurse practitioners. *Journal of Nurse Education*, **19** (1), 41–45

Comer L (1974) *Wedlocked Women*. Leeds: Feminist Books

Coppolillo H (1975) The feminist movement: implications for psychiatry and the family. *Journal of the Tennessee Medical Association*, **68** (7), 536–40

Council for the Education and Training of Health Visitors (1977) *An Investigation into the Principles of Health Visiting*. London: CETHV

Dahl T & Snare A (1978) The coercion of privacy. In Smart B & Smart C eds *Women, Sexuality and Social Control*. London: Routledge & Kegan Paul

Daly M (1978) *Gynecology. The Metaethics of Radical Feminism*. Boston: Beacon Press

Dingwall R (1977) *The Social Organisation of Health Visiting Training*. London: Croom Helm

Du Bois B (1983) Passionate scholarship: notes on values, knowing and method in feminist social science. In Bowles G & Duelli Klein R ed *Theories of Women's Studies*. London: Routledge & Kegan Paul

Evans M (1983) In praise of theory: the case for women's studies. In Bowles G & Duelli Klein R ed *Theories of Women's Studies*. London: Routledge & Kegan Paul

Evason E (1982) *Hidden Violence. Battered Women in Northern Ireland*. Belfast: Farset Co-operative Press

Glass L & Brand K (1975) Perils and parallels of women and nursing. *Nursing Forum*, **14** (2), 160–174

Kent S (1975) Coping with sexual identity crises after mastectomy. *Geriatrics*, **30** (10), 145–146

Kjervik D & Martinson J (1979) *Women in Stress: A nursing perspective*. New York: Appleton-Century-Crofts

Kravetz D & Sargent A (1975) Consciousness raising groups. *Supervisor Nurse* **6** (10), 26–27, 29–31

Krizinofski M (1973) Human sexuality and nursing practice. *Nursing Clinics of North America*, **8** (4), 673–681

Lesson J & Gray J (1978) *Women and Medicine*. London: Tavistock

McKinley J (1970) *Some Aspects of Lower Working Class Utilization Behaviour*. Unpublished PhD thesis, Aberdeen University

Miers M (1979) Health costs of life styles. In Atkinson P, Dingwall R & Murcott A ed *Prospects for the National Health*. London: Croom Helm

Oakley A (1974) *The Sociology of Housework*. Oxford: Martin Robertson

Orr J (1980) *Health Visitor Students' Perceptions of Women*. Unpublished

Orr J (1985) Assessing individuals and families. In Luker K & Orr J eds *Health Visiting*. Oxford: Blackwell

Philips A & Rakusen J (1978) ed *Our Bodies, Ourselves*. Boston Women's Health Collective. Harmondsworth: Penguin

Randolph B *et al* (1979) Consciousness-raising groups. *American Journal of Nursing*, **5**, 922–924

Rich A (1977) *Of Woman Born*. London: Virago

Rimmer L (1983) The economics of work and caring. In Finch J & Groves D ed *A Labour of Love, Women, Work and Caring*. London: Routledge & Kegan Paul

Rossiter C & Wicks M (1982) *Crisis or Challenge? Family Care, Elderly People and Social Policy*. London: Study Commission on the Family

Shockley J (1974) Perspectives in femininity: *Implications for nursing*, **3** (6), 34–40

Spender D (1980) *Man Made Language*. London: Routledge & Kegan Paul

Stark *et al* (1979) *Psychiatric Perspectives on the Abuse of Women*. Centre for Health Studies, Yale University

Tcheng-Laroche *et al* (1979) Middle income divorced female heads of families: their lifestyles, health and stress levels. *Canadian Journal of Psychology*, **24**, 135–142

Thorpe E (1979) A woman's place. *Nursing Times*, **75** (10), 348–349

Urban T (1972) Wives needs as related to the perceptions of their husbands' post mental hospital behaviour. *Community Mental Health Journal*, **8** (12), 120–129

Weingourt R (1979) Battered women and the grieving process *Journal of Psychiatric Nursing*, **17** (4), 40–47

Westkott M (1983) Women's studies as a strategy for change; between criticism and vision. In Bowles G & Duelli Klein R eds *Theories of Women's Studies*. London: Routledge & Kegan Paul

Wilson E (1977) *Women and the Welfare State*. London: Tavistock

6

Women as Gynaecology Patients and Nurses

CHRISTINE WEBB

About the Author

I went into nursing straight from school when I was 18, and five years later I felt I had had enough! My constant physical and emotional exhaustion was due less to the heavy workload than to a realisation that I would probably never be able to exercise any autonomy in my work, and that I had become a rigid and insensitive task-performer instead of a caring nurse.

Leaving nursing – temporarily as it turned out – to become a sociology student in 1968 was a powerful and liberating experience. I was able to analyse and understand better the way I had been socialised as a nurse, and why people working in hospitals behaved in such an oppressive way. Feminism did not become part of this understanding until the early 1970s when, having left university with the somewhat naive belief that I could use my new awareness to change nursing, I got a job as a sister on a gynaecology ward and became involved with a group of women medical workers who wrote health education leaflets for women and supported each other by talking about their working situations and troubles.

Feminism gradually became the most important basis for my work as a nurse and when the chance came to work on a research study looking at recovery from hysterectomy I seized it eagerly. Since then, all my research work and some of my teaching in nursing have concentrated on women's health. Doing this research, both with gynaecology patients and nurses, and experiencing gynaecological treatment as a patient over the past two years have sharpened my belief that feminist ideas have a vast liberating potential for nurses, both women and men. I am convinced that an exploration of feminist writings and participation in groups and campaigns would lead nurses to be able to practise real caring nursing instead of the alienated and subservient forms of 'patient care' they are often involved in at present.

As a teacher on an undergraduate course for nursing students, I am continuing with research into the implications of sexuality and gender for nurses and nursing care.

This chapter tells the story of two research projects – one with women having a hysterectomy and another with gynaecology nurses – and of my own experiences as a gynaecology patient. When I began the study of women going through the process of having a hysterectomy, the first interviews revealed yawning gaps in women's knowledge about the operation. Women had often been informed what treatment they would have without any chance to ask questions, discuss possible alternatives and voice their fears. They had been examined by a nameless doctor in front of a crowd of onlookers who mumbled inaudibly amongst themselves, and were sometimes told bluntly that their symptoms were simply due to anxiety.

When, coincidentally, I became a gynaecology patient while I was in the middle of the research, I had exactly the same experiences and this made me want to look at gynaecology from the point of view of nurses. I wanted to try to understand how women nurses, of whom I am one, made sense of the situation in which they worked and in which they witnessed women being subjected to such apparently insensitive treatment. How did women nurses feel when they watched or participated in these scenes, and how were they as women able to accommodate to this day in, day out demeaning of people like themselves? What marks did it leave on them and why were they unable or unwilling to do anything about it?

Studying hysterectomy patients

My original plan for the hysterectomy study had been to interview 25 women three or four weeks before their operation was scheduled, and then again three months afterwards. Another group of 25 would be interviewed three months afterwards to assess whether being interviewed before operation had had any influence on events. Being interviewed, having someone show enough interest in them to come to their homes and talk to them for an hour or so about their experiences and feelings, could have influenced women's thinking and how they coped, and having the two different groups would allow me to assess this possible influence.

The purpose of the study was to follow up a clue from my earlier research with 142 women who had had a hysterectomy, from which it emerged that very little help had been given to them and little communication had taken place between the women and their partners and families after the operation. From this previous study it appeared that the quality of recovery might be affected by social support, particularly of the emotional kind, so that those with good support might progress more quickly and be happier with their recovery (Webb & Wilson-Barnett 1983). Therefore, I wanted to hear how women prepared for their operation by making plans and talking to people in order to arrange their convalescence, to whom they talked, what kinds of help they felt would be most beneficial, and their expectations of how their needs would be met. Then, at the interview three months after-wards, I was interested to find out whether their expectations had been fulfilled, who had actually given help and support, what forms this had taken, whether unfulfilled hopes had led to disappointment, and whether in the light of experience they would still focus on the same needs or whether different ones had developed. From the study I hoped to learn how health workers, and particularly nurses, could help women to get the kinds of support they wanted and needed.

Although I was a nurse with experience as a gynaecology ward sister and researcher, I had some difficulty getting permission from gynaecologists at the local hospital to interview 'their' patients. They had probably never come across a nurse researcher before, and the usual 'rules' for doctor–nurse encounters came into play. Straightforward requests by letter to the relevant committee, reinforced by talking to the chairmen (sic!), resulted in little progress other than suggestions about how I ought to modify my research design in order to 'improve' it. As a trained and formally qualified researcher, I felt that this advice from people without such training and experience reflected not a scientific interest in rigorous research methods but the tendency of doctors to feel it is appropriate to tell us how to live aspects of our lives which are quite beyond their professional sphere. However, if I wanted to do my study it seemed as if I had no alternative but to play 'the doctor–nurse game' (Stein 1976), and so I went to see one gynaecologist informally and asked him to help me on a personal basis to gain access to patients. He granted me his patronage in response to this approach along the lines recommended by Florence Nightingale herself, who counselled nurses not to con-front doctors directly but to use 'feminine wiles' to get their way. These difficulties in getting the study started weighed heavily on my mind as I did the first interviews and heard what women had to say about their early experiences in out patient clinics when they were put on the waiting list to have a hysterectomy.

Early research experiences

None of the women I contacted showed any reluctance to be interviewed. Quite the contrary, in fact, they were often eagerly awaiting my phone call after receiving an introductory letter explaining about the study. The letter had explained that I was a former gynaecology ward sister who had already completed one research project on recovery from hysterectomy, and therefore I was seen as someone who knew about the process on which women were about to embark.

As I tried to pursue the questions on my interview guide, it soon became obvious that I would get nowhere if I tried to carry on in this way because the women's needs for information were so great that I could not ignore them. Rarely, if ever, had they had the chance to spend as much time as they needed talking with a 'medical expert' and the usual research situation was completely reversed. Instead of the interviewees being a 'captive audience' for my questions, I was a captive nurse to whom they could put all the questions they had about their impending operations. Some of the topics they raised included:

> 'What exactly do they take away?'
> 'How long should I wait for sex afterwards?'
> 'Is sex likely to be any different for us?'
> 'What happens to the sperm then? Where does it go when the
>   womb is gone?'
> 'I think I am going to start my period on the day I am due to go
>   into hospital? What shall I do?'

When I asked women what they had been told at the hospital, they replied:

> 'He didn't explain what the operation might be, and I didn't
>   ask because I'm not shy but there was about 6 students
>   round the bed'.
> 'He just popped in after the student examined me and said I
>   needed a hysterectomy, and that was it. He buzzed off'.

Faced with this situation, I did not feel I could do what research textbooks recommend and reply 'Well that's an interesting question, but right now I'm more interested in what *you* think'. If I had tried to do this, I think the interviews would simply have ground to a halt. Why should the women have given me any information if I refused to take what they said seriously? Furthermore, as a feminist and a nurse with a little experience – soon to be greatly increased – as a patient, it was impossible for me personally to adopt such a strategy.

I was forced by these first few interviews radically to reassess my plans, but I did so with great trepidation because of my earlier contacts with the gynaecologists. One of them had reluctantly agreed to allow the interviews to go ahead as an information-gathering exercise, but no authorisation had been given for me to impart information to the interviewees. If I stepped beyond the boundaries set for me as a nurse researcher by the controlling doctor, would I be accused of encroaching on his professional territory and would the study be halted? I suspected that this could happen, because the women were implicitly – and often explicitly – criticising doctors' treatment of them. Should I go back to the doctor, explain what had happened, and ask his permission to give information at the interview? If I did this and he refused, how would I deal with the knowledge that women's needs were being neglected on such a scale?

My dilemmas were resolved in my own mind after re-reading what other feminist researchers had written about studying women. Ann Oakley (1981) had had similar experiences to mine in her study of motherhood, when her interviewees had been eager to ask her for advice and information because she had had children herself. She too found textbook advice to be not only counterproductive but also a misrepresentation of what really happens in any research interview when women interview other women, but particularly when the interviewer is a feminist. Cautions that interviewers should build up rapport by a few superficial remarks about the weather, and not give away their personal beliefs and opinions, lead to an artificial situation which is so unlike any usual exchange between people that it is nonsense to claim that these strategies increase the validity of the interview as a research tool. This kind of sanitised interview excludes the reality of social life both for the interviewer and the interviewee, and therefore claims of its superior scientific status are unjustified. If we want to know how people feel and what they think, we should ask them in a way which is natural and similar to how we usually learn from others in everyday life, so that they come to trust us because we show interest in what is important to them. Researchers can only do this by entering into the research encounter as people in the same way as they do in everyday social life. They should invest their subjectivity or individuality in the research and make themselves vulnerable in the same way as they ask their interviewees to do. Their work will then be more, not less, rigorous because it places people's experiences and exist-ences firmly within the research and sees their point of view as a legitimate perspective from which to interpret the world (Smith 1979; Roberts 1981).

The 'objective interviewer' stance reflects a male perspective on social life, which needs to be replaced by a sociology for women which is a form of critique going beyond mere criticism to building an alternative (Smith 1979). This sociology for women would recognise that simply adding women in as a topic of study is not enough (Stanley & Wise 1983). We must start in the everyday world of experience and identify women as active agents and not merely as passive objects in research. Instead of suppressing the personal, women's standpoint should be placed firmly on the agenda so that research becomes a cooperative enterprise between the women who are involved both as interviewers and interviewees. Research with and by women can then be a form of consciousness-raising for all, so that everyone involved comes to see reality differently and we begin to develop ways of changing our lives.

My consciousness as a researcher was raised by listening to my interviewees and by re-reading what these feminists had written, and I was convinced that I should change my own approach from one of merely asking questions to one in which I told the hysterectomy patients at the outset that I had come to share with them questions and information. I would ask my questions, they should feel completely free to ask me anything they wished, and I would answer as best I could on the basis of my experience as a nurse who had made a particular study of hysterectomy. I would not do a 'smash and grab raid' (Rapoport & Rapoport 1976), rushing in, seizing data, raising issues in women's minds, and leaving a mess for them to clear up afterwards. We would talk about their concerns and, if I could not help them myself, I would make suggestions about how they might get their problems taken seriously by others. If my strategy was challenged by doctors, I would justify my decisions by explaining why I had chosen this method and why I felt that morally there was no other path open to me.

Often during the interviews done after adopting this new approach, I would spend more time talking than listening to the women. I explained exactly what would be removed when the operation was done, and that the ovaries, vagina and external parts would remain intact. I told women what to expect in hospital as they were prepared for and recovered from the actual surgery, and I described what interviewees in my previous study had said about their progress and how they had felt as they convalesced.

As I spoke, numerous other questions arose for the women and we often had a discussion about topics which do not have an easy answer, such as what causes fibroids, why some women get depressed after having a baby or an operation, and what causes premenstrual tension. Sometimes it seemed appropriate to share with them my own current experiences as a gynaecology patient at another local hospital. I did this to validate their concerns by showing that, even as someone supposedly knowledgeable and experienced in handling the system, I could still feel the same frustrations and distresses as them and not succeed in finding out what I needed to know. These experiences could then be recognised not as resulting from personal inadequacies nor as rare occurrences, but as events that happen to many women and which we need to struggle to change. If I felt that further information or discussion was wanted or needed by women, I would suggest ways of trying to ensure that these were gained. For example, they might telephone the doctor's secretary and ask for an appointment to have a discussion, they could take someone with them on their next visit to boost confidence and help remember all their questions, or they could make a list of questions and use it as a reminder during a consultation. If they felt either that they could not approach a doctor or did not feel clear after talking to him, they might ask a nurse to have a talk with them, or ask her to get the doctor to spend more time discussing their questions. One woman, for example, was concerned that her husband did not understand that she would be unable to carry on with housework as normal when she came out of hospital:

> *Woman*: 'I think it would be useful if someone could talk to the husbands at some time, especially if they are like my husband.'
>
> *CW*: 'If you feel that you would like the sister in the hospital to speak to your husband, just ask and she will be happy to do it for you'.
>
> *Woman*: 'If you think it will be all right – you don't like to use up their time when they have other things that are more important'.

Ways of coping with experiences in hospital frequently cropped up in our discussions. Women were apprehensive about pain or vomiting after the operation, about not being able to use a bedpan, or about bursting their stitches. Again, I gave suggestions of how to manage; for example, I emphasised that pain should be relieved after operations so that patients can relax, breathe adequately, and move around to prevent thromboses in the legs. I advised women to ask nurses for injections or tablets for pain relief as they felt the need, and not to wait for these to be offered or for the drug trolley to come round.

When our discussion seemed to be drawing to a close I always checked to see if women had any further questions and asked them how they felt about my coming to see them. One replied:

> 'I was pleased actually because I got the letter not very long after I had been to the hospital and thought it was a good idea. It gives you a chance to ask questions and find out more about it and not go into it blind or knowing very little'.

Experiencing recovery

At the interviews three months after the operation, when I both re-visited the original 25 women and went for the first time to see 25 others, the same pattern was repeated. The balance of talking between me and the women changed a lot because by now they had gained a great deal of expertise based on their own experiences, but they still had many unanswered questions.

Like those in my earlier study, these women were overwhelmingly glad they had had the operation. When I asked how they felt about having no more periods they replied, 'Smashing! That is one big advantage because I did have terrible times' or 'It doesn't bother me. I've always been used to heavy losses and it's a big change'. Several remarked that they still had premenstrual symptoms and wondered if this was normal. I explained that their ovaries, which produce the hormones leading to the physical symptoms, were still active although there was no more menstruation, and that this would cease at the time of the menopause just as if the women had not had a hysterectomy. On hearing this one woman said:

> 'I thought I was going out of my mind. I wish they had explained that to me. I kept feeling I was going to start, but I thought 'it can't be'.

With regard to not being able to become pregnant, interviewees were again satisfied, saying for example:

> *Woman*: 'Well I couldn't before anyway because I had been sterilised'.
> *CW*: 'Did having the hysterectomy make you think about having babies?'
> *Woman*: 'Oh no!'
>
> *Woman*: 'It doesn't matter. I think I did my share – I had three and that was sufficient.'

CW: 'Did having the operation make you think about it again or not?'
Woman: 'No. I wasn't interested in having any more babies so it never troubled me.'

Lack of information once more emerged as a problem and many women were very critical about this, just as they had been earlier. The following extracts illustrate what they said:

Woman: 'I would have liked a bit more information. Half the problem is worrying about it and not knowing.'

Those who had complications following their operations often said they would have liked to have had warning of possible after-effects so that they would be prepared and not get frightened. One woman put it this way:

Woman: 'I think they should warn you about complications. It would give you some warning so that you know it can happen or it's nothing to worry about'.
CW: 'Do you think that might frighten people?'
Woman: 'I don't see why it should. If somebody had told me that I might see a bit of blood I would not have been so frightened. I thought I was going to have to rush back to the hospital with a haemorrhage. I think they should tell you that you might have a complication or infection or lose a few drops of blood – then you wouldn't worry so much.'

Staff may be reluctant to talk about the possibility of infection, bleeding, and so on, for fear of causing patients unnecessary worry. But patients themselves, both in this study and in my earlier one, said they would rather know what to expect and then if anything did happen they would be more able to cope because it would not be so unexpected. Giving this type of information is useful provided it is accompanied by suggestions of how to manage, such as whether to call a doctor or take any medication, or whether the event is just part of normal recovery and no action is needed.

Women said they had wanted detailed advice about how to build up activities, and that it was not enough simply to be told not to do heavy lifting or to take it easy. Above all, they wanted the advice to be realistic:

Woman: 'The doctor said to me that I would be back at work in six weeks, but in no way could I have gone to work in six weeks. It was ridiculous.'
CW: 'How did you feel about being told that?'
Woman: 'It made me feel guilty. I was made redundant last

year and I have to try and find another job. I know my husband wants me to get a job, so I didn't tell him what the doctor said because I felt so guilty.'

Social support

The subject of my original research proposal was support for women having a hysterectomy, and what they said about lack of information at all stages indicates that this kind of support from hospital staff did not meet their needs. Matching with my earlier study (Webb & Wilson-Barnett 1983), communications among women and their partners and families had been unsatisfactory too. I asked women how their partners felt about their having the operation, and a typical reply would be:

'I don't know. He has never actually said. I don't think he was bothered really.'

Forty of the 50 women in the study had a male partner, and 24 of these did not know his opinion of their operation and recovery. Eight men had indicated positive views and the remaining eight had made negative remarks about the woman's operation and recovery.

Of the total of 50 women interviewed, 20 said they had no particular confidante with whom they could talk over their worries, whether this was their partner, a relative or close friend. Twenty-nine women said their families were sympathetic, but 11 had neither a particular confidante nor a sympathetic family. Of the 25 women interviewed both before and after the operation, nine reported that the help and support they had hoped for had not actually materialised.

When there was someone in whom they could confide, this had been a great source of comfort:

'I think Margaret has been the most helpful because she sits down and has a chat. Not just about the operation, you know, like she sits and has a chat about everything. You need somebody to talk to and she's been great.'

People had often shown their concern for women during recovery by discouraging them from being active and telling them they were doing too much, but this was not appreciated:

CW: 'How did you feel when people said you were doing too much?'
Woman: 'Sort of moody. You can get fed up if people are keeping on at you like that. It gets you down a bit.'

Women wanted to control their own recovery, felt they themselves could understand their own bodies and judge what was appropriate, and wanted to be allowed to do so. Being discouraged from being active made them feel frustrated and even angry.

'Old wives' tales' about hysterectomy were in wide circulation amongst the women and their partners, families and friends. Thirty-eight of the 50 women had heard tales about growing facial hair after a hysterectomy, putting on weight, 'going off sex', being unable to satisfy a male partner sexually, taking a year or more to recover, or getting depressed. These tales, passed on by women from previous generations, recount experiences from a time when anaesthetics were less safe and more physically disturbing to the body, when patients stayed in bed for several weeks after operations, and when surgeons often removed the ovaries with a hysterectomy, thus precipitating women into an immediate menopause instead of a gradual and natural one. So it is not surprising that for our grandmothers hysterectomy was something to be dreaded. Getting over the physical assault and lying around at home, probably feeling isolated and lonely, may indeed have often led to depression.

These stories, then, are based on women's actual experiences and are not the irrational myths which the term 'old wives' tales' is often taken to imply. As women's own experiences change so will the stories they tell, and this is already beginning to happen. Twenty-six of my interviewees had also heard optimistic stories about how well and restored they would feel once they had recovered and no longer had to suffer frequent, continuous or irregular menstrual floodings.

Doctors tell their tales, too, and these gain the status of scientific theory by being published in medical journals. Their articles report varying amounts of depression caused by hysterectomy, although the 'research' is often no more than personal opinions backed up by psychoanalytic ideas about 'castration anxiety' and 'penis envy' among women who, after a hysterectomy, are supposed to become depressed because they are then certain that they can never get a substitute penis by having a male child. 'Psychological outcome' is a main focus of medical research into hysterectomy, but in my previous study those women who were dissatisfied with their recovery put this down to physical and not psychological complications, particularly infections of the wound, vagina and urinary tract. Levels of depression have recently been shown by several sound studies to *fall* as women recover (Gath 1980; Coppen *et al.* 1981). Since infections after operation are iatrogenic, or caused by the treatment, it seems that doctors preferred to concentrate on stereotyped conceptions of women as emotional and ruled by their reproductive organs rather than draw attention to their own deficiencies. As women are increasingly realising, 'old wives' tales' usually have a validity based on women's actual life experiences, whereas 'old doctors' tales' often appear more like myths and fantasies (Ehrenreich & English 1979; Versluysen 1980).

Women in my study who had a job outside the home had talked more to other women about their operation and had heard more positive stories. Having an outside job seemed to be important for recovery, just as it has been found in other studies to help prevent depression and feelings of isolation and frustration (Brown & Harris 1978; Hobson 1978). Women who were full-time house-wives were very much more likely to say that their families and friends were unsympathetic. This might be either because their isolation allowed them less contact with people who could be supportive or because they were felt by others to need less help because they were 'not working', housework being seen as a woman's natural and normal role and not as a real job requiring long working hours and great physical stamina. Those with sympathetic families, on the other hand, were less likely to say they were still suffering from tiredness three months after their operation, possibly not only because they received more help but also because their families' interest and concern helped them to cope emotionally with their recovery.

At the end of all the interviews I asked women to complete a short pencil and paper test called a Mood Adjective Checklist (Lishman 1972) to assess levels of anxiety, depression, fatigue, hostility and vigour. Those who had done the test twice, at the pre- and post-operative interviews, were less anxious, depressed, hostile and fatigued, and more vigorous three months after their operation than before. Although the second group had only done the test at the follow-up interview, they did not differ on any important biographic details (age, social class, family size, medical history, etc) from the two-interview group, so it is possible to compare their scores on the test. Comparing the two groups in this way, those who had had the pre-operative discussion with me had better scores on all the measures, but a particularly interesting difference occurred with the hostility score. The one-visit group had significantly higher levels of hostility, perhaps because they were dissatisfied with the levels of information they had received about their hysterectomy and convalescence.

The only other statistically significant difference between the two groups three months after operation was that, although 24 out of the total 50 had voiced some criticism of their treatment, those whom I had visited were more critical. A possible interpretation of this is that, having discussed with me what was involved and what treatment to expect, their hopes were raised and they were then disappointed and more critical when things did not work out as they had hoped. By sharing my knowledge with them I had raised their expectations and they may have assessed their experiences in a different light.

Personal experiences of being a gynaecology patient

I, too, was critical of the way I was treated as a gynaecology patient, both in an outpatient clinic and in a ward. When I had a treatment performed in the clinic to 'freeze' a cervical erosion, I had a strong physical reaction, with pain, palpitations and a vivid red flushing of the skin from my chest upwards. I was told that this was a purely psychological reaction and that the procedure was painless. Later, when I went into the hospital for an overnight stay and further tests, I was seen by four different doctors within the space of less than 24 hours. Each of them addressed me as 'Mrs Er...' as he picked up my notes without stopping actually to read my name and started to try to figure out what to say to me. After the tests, I was told I had endometriosis and was given hormone tablets: my questions about side-effects were brushed aside with brief 'reassurance' that these would only be trivial and transitory. After a few weeks I felt that my whole body had changed and was out of my control, and I was particularly upset to be gaining weight very rapidly despite eating very little. I gained a stone in six weeks and had to buy new trousers because I could no longer fasten the waist of my present ones. The clinic doctor was unable to say whether this was a temporary gain due to fluid retention or a permanent building up of body tissue, but he dismissed my concern by saying that he had no sympathy because his own weight problems were greater than mine.

My own experiences were like a caricature of the sexist male expert doctor putting down the emotional woman. Despite being an experienced nurse and a fairly confident woman in other realms of my life, I was reduced to feeling inadequate, a person who could not be talked to on an equal basis by doctors, and someone whose worries and distress were of no importance.

I remembered from the time I worked on the wards as a nurse that I had also had a great deal of difficulty in being assertive with doctors, both when I wanted to get them to listen to my observations and suggestions and when I felt they were not treating patients as they should. Leaving bedside nursing and going into teaching had allowed me to avoid some of these experiences.

How did women nurses cope when they could not avoid being confronted with this kind of treatment of women patients on an unremitting basis? To try to answer this question, I carried out another study – this time of 30 trained nurses working on gynaecology wards.

Being a gynaecology nurse

Being a gynaecology nurse was both a rewarding and stressful job for the nurses I studied. As I listened and tape-recorded, they told me what they felt were the special needs of the patients they nursed in this speciality where all nurses and patients are women but the majority of doctors are men.

Nurses felt that women were particularly sensitive about disorders of their reproductive systems, and that they had different worries from patients on other wards. As women themselves, nurses felt they could understand and respond to their needs because, even if they had not suffered from the same conditions, they could readily empathise with their patients. They felt that the main and distinctive feature of gynaecology nursing was the amount of time spent just talking to patients, who often had fears of 'losing their womanhood' as a result of having a hysterectomy, for example. I asked the nurses what they told a woman who was about to go home after this operation, and they mentioned the same snippets of information that the patients themselves had done – take it easy, don't do any heavy lifting, and so on. Despite their earlier remarks about 'womanhood', however, no nurse said she would talk about resuming sexual intercourse nor any other aspect of femininity. Indeed, they found difficulty in explaining what was meant by 'womanhood' or 'femininity', and answered in terms such as:

> 'I think that is a bit hard to say really. If you have part of your stomach taken away that is a big thing because you have got to have a special diet, watch what you eat. Whereas when you are having a hysterectomy and you won't have any periods any more, again you are just taking away the reproductive system which you are born with and now you just haven't got.'

When we talked about giving 'psychological support' to their patients, too, nurses frequently revealed that they had difficulties with this, none having had any special preparation for their work. Two of the 30 had had a one-hour session on communications skills in their basic training, and one had trained as a psychiatric nurse and this course had included some social skills work. Learning by trial and error and by observing more experienced nurses who had gone through the same process had led to embarrassing situations for many of the nurses, and several were critical of the inadequacy of their training and the kind of care patients received as a result. One said:

> 'I think it's a shame that we can't give them enough of what they feel they obviously need. If they feel the need to form groups (like the Endometriosis Support Group) then it's because we haven't given them enough support or advice, and because of that they have to go to others.'

The principal source of conflict and stress for the majority, 19 of the 30 nurses, was their work with women having abortions. Late terminations of pregnancy (TOP) using an injection into the womb to stimulate abortion were particularly distressing, of course, but sometimes nurses felt that the unpleasantness and pain women experienced would teach them a valuable lesson:

> 'I don't like prostaglandins terminations. I think they should be a very good way of deterring girls especially from making the same mistake again... I feel there is enough education about contraception today for them to have the sense to do something about it.'

Contrary to what they had said about their other patients, nurses had little or no sympathy for TOP patients, and felt they were 'brazen little madams' who boasted to other patients about having an abortion. They were said not to be upset by their situation, but to regard abortion simply as a method of contraception when they 'couldn't be bothered' to use other methods. Nurses were particularly shocked and disapproving of young girls having abortions, and believed that many 15 and 16-year-olds came back several times for repeat abortions.

Women who want an abortion often have great difficulty arranging it. Less than half of abortions are done by the National Health Service and in some areas the figures are much lower (OPCS 1982). Administrative delays or just plain obstructive tactics by professionals cause a great deal of distress and account for some of the later terminations which patients and nurses both find so upsetting. There is no evidence that women simply use abortion instead of contraception, and much evidence that they find it an emotionally traumatic and lonely process which is nevertheless the right decision for them at that time. Use of contraception increases after TOP, and women say the experience gives them greater self-understanding and determination to take more control of their lives in future (Cvejic *et al.* 1977; Freeman 1978).

The nurses interviewed knew little or nothing about abortion patients, their personal and social histories, and why they wanted an abortion. Their medical notes were often skimpy, leaving nurses with the impression that it is very easy to get an abortion and that in fact they are done more or less 'on demand'. Patients came into hospital one day, had the termination the next, and went home on the third day, having had no counselling, with no follow-up planned, and with one pack of oral contraceptive pills or an intra-uterine contraceptive device (IUD) which had been fitted at the time of the operation. Nurses were simply required to 'process' them, had no chance to get to know them as individuals, and felt they had no special role in their care. So when these women were admitted in a highly emotional state, often having battled to get the service they so desperately wanted, and nurses felt they were merely carrying out doctors' arbitrary decisions, it is easy to understand how women on both sides of the abortion encounter can feel unhappy and abused.

Nurses spoke well of the mainly male doctors they worked with, saying that patients wanted a doctor who was good at the job and had no particular preference for a woman doctor. However, many nurses recounted incidents like the following, in which they felt that men doctors had humiliated women patients or not taken their problems seriously.

> 'Some doctors don't really want to know. They say what they have to say, but they don't really sit down and have a good talk with them, not unless they really have to. Take heavy bleeding, for example. It's something they deal with every day and they just pass it off as a normal thing.'

Some felt strongly about this, but helpless to deal with the situation. A nurse who had tried to draw doctors' attention to their behaviour had received in return the suggestion that *she* had a problem:

> 'I think we should have some form of body where we could go and report things like that. I know we can say to the doctor, "I thought you were a bit unfair to her", but they just laugh and say, "What's wrong with you today?"'

Being a gynaecology nurse was clearly a very emotionally stressful, as well as a rewarding, job for these women. This was confirmed, I feel, by the fact that they spoke very easily and openly of their deepest feelings about their work and their patients. Some of them knew me slightly because I supervised student nurses or came and spoke to some of my hysterectomy study recruits on their wards. But most were meeting me for the first time when I approached them to ask them to take part in the research. In some ways they might have been suspicious of me because I was a relatively high status nurse teaching at a university and had been given permission to do the study by their nurse managers. The fact that, despite these constraints, they shared so much with me suggests that their own needs for support were not being met in the work situation and that, when I offered a chance to release these feelings they had been holding back, a stream of distress bubbled out.

In that sense, perhaps I gave something to the nurses in return for the time and attention they gave to me. I also sent each of them a copy of my research report, and some contacted me later to discuss it. At first they were very upset to read what was written, while recognising that they were their own words that were being given back to them. But later they contacted me again to say that they had thought over the report and decided to ask their nurse managers to provide counselling and communications skills training for them so that they could try to fulfil this part of their role better. I appreciated their telling me this because listening to them talking and re-playing the tapes had been a moving and distressing experience for me as I heard them talking about how they and their patients were controlled and put down by the male-dominated 'health' system which inhibits women nurses and patients from sharing their knowledge and problems and acting together to change things for themselves.

What I have learned from the research

Talking to women patients has taught me that women want and need nurses to give them a great deal of detailed information about how their bodies work, and how they can expect treatments to affect their physical and emotional health, their family and working lives. Telling them simply to take things easy is not helpful because it is too vague and, for many women who will receive very limited help at home, it is annoying because it is unrealistic for them and can make them feel guilty that they are not doing 'the right thing'.

Nurses may need to talk to partners and families, too, explaining how women will feel, what activities are advisable, and what assistance is needed. Talking to women themselves alone and together with their families helps them to feel that their concerns are important and that people have the time and interest to take them seriously, and it will begin a process of opening up about and sharing feelings which women told me was valuable as they coped with recovery. Families and friends may need advice about giving time for women just to talk about their experiences, and how to be most supportive – for example, the hysterectomy patients did not want to be overprotected and discouraged from doing things. They wanted people to allow them to trust their own judgement as they began to regain independence and get back to normal life.

The women I interviewed needed an individual space to talk to someone who could give them realistic information and advice, but nurses also told me how much their patients discussed among themselves in the ward. This gives nurses an opportunity to bring women together to share their worries and give each other mutual support by acknowledging shared concerns. Many patients would welcome written information, too, and nurses could write leaflets for them to take away and consult later to refresh their memories, and to show to their partners and families when they are attempting to arrange help and support at home.

Helping women to gain knowledge and understand anatomical and technical terms gives them more confidence to ask for information, and as well as this nurses can arrange opportunities for patients to have time with doctors, staying with them if they would like support of this kind. Nurses can initiate discussions with doctors in patients' presence if they know that women would like to talk about a particular issue but are reluctant to raise it themselves.

Doing these research projects, talking to these women patients and nurses, and being a patient myself have strongly reinforced my belief that feminist ideas could be very important for nursing in many ways. By sharing knowledge with patients in a mutual exchange and non-hierarchical relationship, nurses could help patients to take control of their own bodies and their medical encounters. By the same process, nurses themselves could learn more about their patients' experiences and be able to pass on this knowledge to other women, but they could also gain a lot for themselves. The relationships built up with patients would add to nurses' own self-esteem because this would be a distinctive contribution they as women nurses would be making to the quality of their patients' care. Nurses themselves could gain as well as give emotional support in this way, and by extending this sharing of knowledge and feelings with others, they could build the strength to take on bigger struggles.

I feel that if women nurses and patients could come to share in this way, to explode myths about what 'scientific medicine' has to say about women, and to refuse to accept demeaning behaviour from doctors, then they could together be a tremendous force for change in health care.

Jo Ann Ashley, an American feminist nurse, has pointed out that traditional professionalism in nursing has made us 'split ourselves off from the common life of women and deny our female heritage and identity in our work' (Ashley 1980: 19). She believes that often women risk their health by going to male professionals, whose working model emphasises rationality, non-emotionality and obedience to a father-figure represented by the male doctor. In the past, nurses have acted as advocates for doctors, but she would like to see women nurses rejecting these professional values which are hostile towards women. In asserting that 'women nurses are *women* first' (Ashley 1980: 21. Emphasis in the original) she hopes that nurses can become advocates of women, explaining the risks of treatment, helping them to find competent and reliable practitioners, and standing by other women, both patients and colleagues, to establish a 'community of shared caring'.

Acknowledgements

I would like to thank all the women who participated in my research and shared their insights and feelings with me. Without them I would, of course, have been unable to write this chapter. But also I would have been deprived of many opportunities to think about, and try to understand more clearly, our struggles as women and nurses to achieve the kind of health care we need.

References

Ashley J A (1980) Power in structured misogyny: implications for the politics of care. *Advances in Nursing Science*, **2** (3), 3–22
Brown GW & Harris T (1978) *Social Origins of Depression*. London: Tavistock Publications

Coppen A, Bishop M, Beard RJ, Barnard GJR & Collins (1981) Hysterectomy, hormones and behaviour. *Lancet*, **i**, 126–128

Cvejic H, Lipper I, Kinch RA & Benjamin P (1977) Follow-up of 50 adolescent girls 2 years after abortion. *Canadian Medical Association Journal*, **116** (1), 44–46

Ehrenreich B & English E (1979) *For Her Own Good, 150 Years of the Experts' Advice to Women*. London: Pluto Press

Freeman EW (1978) Abortion: subjective attitudes and feelings. *Family Planning Perspectives*, **10** (3), 150–155

Gath D (1980) Psychiatric aspects of hysterectomy. In Robins L, Clayton P & Wing J ed *The Social Consequences of Psychiatric Illness*. New York: Bruner-Mazel

Hobson D (1978) Housewives: isolation as oppression. In Women's Studies Group, Centre for Contemporary Cultural Studies, Birmingham ed, *Women Take Issue*. London: Hutchinson

Lishman WA (1972) Selective factors in memory. Part 2: Affective disorders. *Psychological Medicine*, **2**, 248–253

Oakley A (1981) *Subject Women*. Glasgow: Fontana

Office of Population Censuses & Surveys (1982) *1980 Abortion Statistics*. Series AB No. 7. London: HMSO

Rapoport R & Rapoport RN (1976) *Dual-career Families Re-examined*. London: Martin Robinson

Roberts H ed (1981) *Doing Feminist Research*. London: Routledge & Kegan Paul

Smith DE (1979) A sociology for women. In Sherman JA & Beck ET ed *The Prism of Sex*. Madison: University of Wisconsin Press

Stanley L & Wise S (1983) *Breaking Out: Feminist Consciousness and Feminist Research*. London: Routledge & Kegan Paul

Stein L (1976) The doctor–nurse game. *Archives of General Psychiatry*, **16**, 699–703

Versluysen MC (1980) Old wives' tales? Women Healers in English history. In Davies C ed *Rewriting Nursing History*. London: Croom Helm

Webb C & Wilson Barnett J (1983) Coping with hysterectomy. *Journal of Advanced Nursing*, **8** (3), 311–319

7

A Feminist Approach to General Practice

MAGGIE EISNER   MAUREEN WRIGHT

About the Authors

Maureen Wright

I would not have become a doctor without the support of my childhood GP. When I was eight, I was talking to him about my ambition to become a nurse and he said, 'Why not be a doctor? You'll enjoy it more.'

I found medical training an isolating experience, not only because I am a woman, but also because, unlike most medical students, I come from a non-professional, lower-middle-class family. When I qualified, my first reaction was relief that I now had the means to support myself and any children that I might have – the first time that I had consciously seen this as a motive for my choice.

After qualification, I dealt with my ambivalence towards medicine by spending six months working the hundred-hour week of a junior hospital doctor followed by six months living off my savings and forgetting I was a doctor. By then it was the mid-1970s: I was living in a large squat in London, going to my first women's meetings and becoming involved in community politics.

I became a GP sooner than I planned: I went to help at a collective practice in London for six weeks and stayed for four years. Having learned general practice within an unconventional setting, I am now struggling to become effective in a conventional practice. I work in a long-established health centre practice in Bristol with three full-time male partners. It's a typical 'part-time lady doctor job' and its limitations reflect the reality of being a single woman with two small children (aged six and three) as well as being a GP.

Maggie Eisner

I cannot imagine a job which I would enjoy more than being a GP. My mother, a doctor, encouraged me to study medicine because she viewed it as both useful

113

to society and a sensible career offering secure employment and financial independence. I chose general practice to escape the impersonal, hierarchical hospital world, and so that I could be involved with a wide variety of people, health problems and situations, following people's changing lives over long periods.

I spent four years dividing my time between part-time jobs in two contrasting South London practices: one, in an inner-city area, was a conventional group practice dominated by the senior partner; the other was run as a collective, based on socialist and feminist ideas.

During this period, there were two major outside influences on my work. The Politics of Health Group helped me to understand how social and political factors are overwhelmingly important in health. An evening course at the Pellin Therapy Centre helped me with my personal development and filled a big gap in my medical training: I learned some invaluable practical ways to help other people with emotional and social difficulties.

I now work full-time in Shipley, Yorkshire, in a Health Centre where there are three separate practices. My predecessor was an elderly man who had practised single-handed; I took over his practice on the same basis, but was joined by a partner after six months. I have no children, and would not have considered even six months' single-handed practice if I had.

Writing together

We have been friends for at least ten years, and used to work together. We now live 200 miles apart and have enjoyed having an excuse to spend weekends writing together. After planning the chapter, we wrote separate versions which we then merged. Fortunately we agreed about what we wanted to say, so have been able to use 'we' throughout the main text. We have included some anecdotes from our individual experiences, and these are printed in small type.

THE CONTEXT OF OUR WORK

Background information

General practice occupies a peculiar position in the Health Service; this section provides some background information to help readers to make sense of what follows.

GPs are not employees of the NHS. Each practice is a small business run by the doctors, who have a contract with the Family Practitioner Committee to provide medical services for the people on their list of patients. We are paid an allowance for running the practice, an annual fee per patient, and additional fees for particular services such as maternity care and contraception. Our total income is meant to cover both our salaries and the expenses of running the practice – in other words, as long as we provide the basic services, we can choose how to spend the money, as well as choosing our own working hours, staff and premises (which we may own, or rent either privately or, in the case of Health Centres, from the Health Authority).

This means that the service someone gets from a GP will depend on that doctor's priorities, and partly explains why the standard of general practice is so variable. It also means that the state has less direct control over GPs than over the doctors it employs directly, who work in hospitals or in community clinics. And as bosses of small businesses, we are also the employers of the receptionists, secretaries and practice nurses we work with (though not of district nurses, health visitors or midwives, who are NHS employees).

GPs can choose to work alone, but most now work in partnerships or larger groups. Single-handed practice provides a very personal service for the patients, but a doctor working alone can usually offer a narrower range of services than a group practice; the doctor often also becomes isolated and idiosyncratic. In a group practice, the doctors may be equal partners and take equal shares of responsibility, work and money, or there may be a hierarchy among them, with a senior partner, and perhaps one or more part-time partners with limited responsibility. The latter are usually women.

The traditional image of the GP as paternalistic, authoritarian and working in isolation has been changing in recent years. The progressive face of general practice is represented by the Royal College of General Practitioners, a body set up along the lines of those governing and setting standards in other medical specialities such as surgery. It was instrumental in developing specialised training for newly qualified doctors wishing to become GPs, and this is now compulsory. The training schemes vary in different areas of the country but all consists of two years' hospital training and a year's apprenticeship with an experienced GP 'trainer'. Throughout, trainees may attend a half-day release course which provides a forum for discussion of problems and issues in general practice, and often some training in counselling and interpersonal skills, which are covered very inadequately at medical school. Almost 50 per cent of GP trainees are now women, but the vast majority of trainers are men.

Some of the ideas in general practice training have considerable appeal: for example, trainees are taught to make diagnoses in every case in 'physical, psychological and social terms'. But women sometimes complain that this approach leads doctors to over-emphasise psychological and social factors in their illnesses. And the Royal College always sees GPs as family doctors; the traditional role of women in society is rarely questioned.

GPs are now seen as specialists, and it is recognised that our relationships with people who consult us are different from those of hospital doctors. Our contact is more intimate and longer-term and our work is much more about caring and reassurance, and less about medical diagnosis and treatment, than most people think.

> My own trainer once said to me 'I think our role is to be the patient's friend'. John Berger's book *A Fortunate Man* (1976) also gives an insight into the close relationships involved in good traditional general practice.

Despite the existence of an influential liberal current, the majority of general practitioners are extremely conservative. For example, 'lady doctors' are not expected to wear trousers at work, and even reading *The Guardian* is enough to earn us the reputation of dangerous radicalism. Our personal lives are assumed to be very conventional indeed:

> I was recently chatting to one of the other Health Centre GPs, who knows I am not married, about a visit to the theatre. When I said 'and we had a drink in the interval', he responded with 'Oh! You said 'we' – are you engaged?'

The basic contradiction

Becoming a feminist and a GP has been, for both of us, a process of putting together brief flashes of insight and puzzling contradictions which have occurred at intervals ever since we first thought of becoming doctors. We have only learned as we went along that the things which attracted us to general practice – autonomy, a relative lack of a hierarchical institution, long-term relationships with many different people – were also the symptoms and results of the enormous privilege and power enjoyed by GPs: we have a lot more money, status and independence than most women. Our feminism has developed from a simple attempt to have straightforward, supportive and honest relationships with the women with whom we work, to include a much more complex understanding of the power relations in our male-dominated, class-ridden society, where doctors (and we must include ourselves) represent a significant area of control over women's lives.

While we were planning this chapter, we spent most of our time discussing the anomaly of being both a feminist and a privileged professional. A useful article by Mary Howell (1979) lists four areas in which the professionalism we absorb with our medical training is in conflict with feminist values:

1   Professionals learn to be arrogant and disrespectful towards people assumed to be less important than ourselves (eg. patients, receptionists, nurses).
2   It is assumed that as professionals, we deserve our privileges (eg. our high incomes, which enable us to pay for other women to clean our houses).
3   Professionals believe that the knowledge and skill we have acquired entitle us to exert control over other people's lives. This also implies keeping our knowledge secret and mysterious.
4   Professionalism defines what is important, valid and scientific (eg. which therapies are acceptable and which 'fringe'; which patients have 'real' diseases and which are wasting the doctor's valuable time).

Trying to get our brains (and especially our consciences) around these contradictions could paralyse us and make it impossible to work at all. Ignoring the contradictions is impossible unless we stop being either feminists or doctors. In our day to day work we inevitably make compromises which make us feel either that we are not being good feminists or that we are not being good doctors. It is easy to feel caught between criticisms from both sides, and end up hurt and vulnerable, or angry and resentful.

So what are we trying to do as feminist GPs? We want to be responsible to the people who come to us for medical help, not a part of the system which oppresses them. We would like to feel we are helping women to take more control over their health, as part of taking more control over their lives. We do not see health as an end in itself, but as a means to a life in which one has the chance to fufil one's potential. We want this for everyone, but as feminists we feel a special responsibility towards women.

Relationships with our fellow-workers

Doctors are notorious for acting in an authoritarian, high-handed way with receptionists, nurses, midwives and other health workers seen as their subordinates.

We need to find ways to counteract our training and learn to respect other health workers as equals, paying constant attention to appreciating their skills, the personal qualities they bring to their work, and the particular problems of their position.

'Progressive' modern general practice emphasises the primary health care team consisting of GPs, health visitors, community nurses, midwives and perhaps social workers (all professionals – receptionists are not even mentioned). Unfortunately the reality is often a hierarchy with GPs at the top, expecting the other members of the team to provide 'handmaiden' support like that received by their hospital colleagues. GPs often talk about the team approach in terms of 'delegating' and reducing their own workload, rather than as a way of enriching everybody's working life and offering a better service. For example, they sometimes query whether a practice nurse could be 'trusted' to take cervical smears, a procedure which is traditionally carried out by doctors. Such a hierarchical view of working relationships obscures the enormous amount the doctors learn from others: knowledge flows up the power pyramid. Many individual GPs do acknowledge this, but it is not recognised in the structure of the team.

In general practice, the doctor is often the employer of the receptionists and possibly other staff. How can we develop democratic working relationships in such a hierarchical structure? We cannot be equal with someone whom we have the power to hire and fire. The present structure of general practice leaves us no choice about this position – we are the employers, and have a responsibility to be good ones. We also need to appreciate that the receptionists are aware of their position as employees.

> Although in our practice I think we all feel like friends, I sometimes notice one of the receptionists looks anxious if I suggest we should have a practice meeting. Her previous experience as an employee leads her to expect a meeting to mean a telling-off from her employer, rather than an opportunity for us all to discuss things as equals.

A receptionist's job is a balancing act between the requirements of the patients and those of the doctor. If receptionists can get close to patients, people benefit from their help and this makes their work more satisfying, but the physical structure of their working environment often makes this impossible. It is hard to make a fruitful relationship through a shatterproof glass partition in a crowded waiting room. The patients may feel that their needs are overwhelmingly urgent and see the receptionist as an irritating barrier between themselves and the doctor; the receptionist must respond to those needs and minimise the irritation while also keeping the doctor happy: this may mean obeying a doctor whom she fears, protecting a tired, overworked doctor of whom she is fond, or even trying to respond to conflicting instructions from different doctors.

> A few months ago, my partner and I appointed two new receptionists; recently they both told me that when they first started, they were more worried about when to bring the doctors their tea than about how to deal with an anxious member of the public or a medical emergency.

Yet receptionists get almost no recognition or support – even basic training is a recent innovation, and few of them have access to it. It is a job where the responsibility is huge, but the power and freedom of action to deal with the responsibility are negligible.

As feminists, our aim is to work on an equal basis with other members of the team – but respecting their skills does not just mean 'You know what you're doing: just get on and do it' because we also have a responsibility to give them support. On the other hand, our feminist position cannot allow us to support other women workers uncritically: it is very difficult for a feminist to work with, for example, a health visitor or midwife who is prejudiced and patronising towards unsupported mothers. If we criticise our colleagues in situations like this, we must try to do it in a sisterly and constructive way, but be aware that we are likely to be seen as exercising our authority as doctors, and resented for it.

As well as trying to establish good relationships on the individual level, we believe it is important to support other women health workers as a group. The health service trades unions have many shortcomings, mirroring some of the faults of the NHS in their hierarchical organisation, with a majority of women at the bottom and men at the top, and in their narrow definition of health and health care. The relative isolation of general practice (even in health centres) can make trades union activity seem irrelevant, and many of the health workers in primary care are not unionised. But the unions do represent the most unified force for defence of the NHS and the jobs of its workers, and perhaps even for progressive changes within it; the women in the health unions deserve the support of feminist doctors.

Sexism in the medical profession

Within the profession the problems facing women GPs are no different from those facing any woman in a man's world: achieving a balance between showing 'we're as good as the men' and changing the definition of 'good'. Although over 80 per cent of GPs are men, women GPs are apparently well accepted. Many group practices consider it useful to have a female partner, who often works on a part-time basis and may be excused on-call duty at nights and weekends. The emphasis in her job is often on women's and children's health: at one level this is a valid response to the demands of women for the choice to see a woman doctor, and it provides fulfilling work for a feminist.

On the other hand the 'lady doctor' is frequently a second-class citizen among the doctors in the practice: she may be exploited financially and her domestic commitments, even if they exist only as a future possibility in her partners' minds, may be used as an excuse to exclude her from decision-making amongst the partners. She also misses the opportunity to use the full range of her skills, and being on call, although burdensome, is also a very special part of general practice, seeing people in their own homes at times of crisis. Moving from a part-time to a full-time partnership, if another partner leaves or retires, may be the easiest route to a full-time partnership for a woman. Medicine, like the other professions, has a place for women – provided the women know their place.

When practices advertise for a full-time partner, what they generally want is not only a man, but a married man whose wife provides a devoted, unpaid back-up service. The doctor's wife answers the telephone, makes meals available at odd and variable times to fit in with the doctor's unpredictable timetable, and provides a lot of emotional support because the doctor is inevitably drained by caring for his patients. A full-time woman GP must make her own arrangements – and we have not even mentioned child care.

So pervasive is the male tradition in medicine that it is easy to forget that there are increasing numbers of women in medicine and that, although our training may teach us to act like men, most of us do identify with other women. Looking for sisterhood in our professional lives can be a way to rally the support of women doctors (including those who do not see themselves as feminists), for a different way of looking at medicine.

I once went with two other feminist doctors to a local GP meeting about rape. Initially, the reaction to the male speaker was a great deal of sniggering and misogynist 'joking' from the male doctors present. When the three of us confronted them with this behaviour, it allowed the few other women present to voice their feelings and fears about rape – especially our vulnerability when visiting patients at night.

What is the best strategy for influencing other doctors? We often feel that we do not fit in at all in medical meetings, and it is easy to be marginalised as eccentrics if we express our ideas too freely. Camouflaging ourselves with conventional clothes and attitudes does not change anything and also puts us at risk of devaluing our feminist principles. One tactic for dealing with this is to keep a low profile until we have established our credibility, and then express our own ideas.

It can be hard to maintain the low profile in the face of such comments as 'but women's position in society isn't a political matter'. My façade was shattered, before I had time to phrase a more diplomatic response, by my impulsive retort 'I've got news for you'. Some progress can be made, though: at the local GP training course, a speaker had said that women ask their GPs for more emotional support than men do, implying that women, being weaker than men, have a greater need for such support. I pointed out that women spend a lot of their time and energy giving emotional support to many people in their lives, and often have no-one but the GP to turn to for their own emotional support. A respected male colleague, sitting behind me, murmured, 'That's a good point'. I was surprised that it seemed to be a new idea to him, but pleased that he did, at least, accept the truth of it.

The need to maintain our credibility with the medical profession can come between us and the people who seek our help.

At a recent home delivery, the birth was imminent when the baby's heart began to show signs of strain by beating more slowly. The midwife and I felt we might need to transfer her to the hospital for a forceps delivery. It is only a five-minute journey and I had few fears for the baby's well-being, but I felt very worried about my reputation with the local obstetric consultants, because I would have to admit that I had gone against accepted medical practice by agreeing to the woman's request that her first baby be born at home. (In fact, the 8lb baby girl was born, healthy and alert, at home before the ambulance arrived).

As isolated GPs, it is extremely difficult for us to influence the way in which our colleagues (even including our own partners) behave to patients or other health workers, and teaching may be a potentially more rewarding area. Students and trainees can sit in on our consultations and have a chance to see the way we relate to the people who consult us, and judge for themselves the value of a 'feminist' way of working. This is much more likely to convince them than the angry interjections we find so hard to suppress at meetings.

The women's health movement

Many feminists would say that it is pointless to try to influence individual doctors in an attempt to change the treatment of women by the medical profession as a whole. Certainly, it is pressure from the outside which has brought about most changes in medical practice – the recent trend away from routine high technology maternity care is an obvious example.

Knowing this, we have both been involved in various groups within the women's health movement. We came to them accustomed to praise and a warm feeling of self-satisfaction as doctors who worked in a more sisterly way than most. It came as a shock, therefore, to discover that feminists saw us as representatives of the very profession from which we felt so different. It was hard to face the uncomfortable truth that, in some ways, we inevitably act like arrogant and insensitive professionals. Our training not only accustoms us to taking a lead and being listened to, so that we intimidate less articulate women, but also gives our contributions the weight of professional opinions, when in reality they may be only personal experiences.

But it is a challenge to act as a resource for groups without using our status as experts to provide answers and control the outcome of discussions. Sharing information without passing on the assumptions and values which we absorbed with it means facing up to the disturbing fact that a lot of professional practice is based on myth and tradition with as little (or less) validity as the 'old wives' tales' which the medical profession disparages (see Chapter 6, Chamberlain (1981) and Ehrenreich & English (1979)).

We have learnt that feminism demands a new approach, not only to the way we practise, but also to the 'scientific facts' on which our knowledge is based. We have had to reassess critically whether there is any scientific basis to the medicine we practise, and the significance of science relative to individual experience (our own and other women's) and to our social and political environment. In our eagerness to purge ourselves of our expert status, we should not go to the other extreme and insist that we have nothing of value to offer.

> I have been invited to speak at several meetings of different groups of women discussing the menopause. Everyone soon realises that the women in the room (often 20 or more) have between them an enormous fund of direct knowledge of the menopause, but maybe I can tell them a bit about what doctors say about it, and pass on experiences from women who have consulted me as patients.

Another way in which we can be useful is in giving practical support to feminist initiatives, such as setting up women's refuges and Rape Crisis Centres. Applications for funding and premises may be more credible if a doctor is on the management group. Once centres are in operation, we can act as informal advisers if we are asked by the women involved. We are interested, too, in the development of feminist Well Woman Centres. It is, however, increasingly clear that these need to be quite different from Well Woman Clinics which replicate conventional medical institutions, and it may be more appropriate for us to offer quiet support than to take a leading role. (This issue is discussed fully in Lisa Saffron's article (Saffron 1985).) We have also found that being part of campaigning groups like the National Abortion Campaign minimises the difficulties of our position. Professional status is irrelevant to much of the work such as duplicating leaflets or organising meetings and we can participate on an equal basis with less temptation to become 'experts with the answers' in discussion and planning.

Although we both became involved with the women's health movement because we felt that we had something to offer, we now know that our contribution has been much smaller than their contribution to our continuing education. Medical training has narrowed our vision: we need the broader vision of the women's movement.

An alternative structure

We worked together for four years in a collective general practice in inner London, which was a conscious attempt to set up an alternative to conventionally organised practice. The experiment ended in 1984 (well after both of us had left) with a bitter dispute between one of the doctors and the rest of the workers at the practice. This painful end of a very important part of our working lives has made it difficult for us to write this section; we have chosen to present a brief description of the practice and then concentrate on what we have learnt from the experience of working there.

The collective included a majority of women; not all of them described themselves as feminists, but feminist principles under-pinned the relations between workers, patients and other people and institutions. There were several general workers who did reception duties, but who also developed relationships with patients which were explicitly recognised by us all as important, nourishing and healing. They suggested and initiated ways of dealing with patients' problems and also learned some basic medical skills like syringing ears and taking cervical smears – this helped to take some of the mystery out of the doctors' tasks. The collective also included acupuncturists, psychotherapists, and women who had learnt health care skills within the women's health movement, in addition to the doctors. We tailored the practice finances to pay all the workers at an equal hourly rate. All of us worked part-time.

We constructed a two-tier decision-making structure in the prac-tice: all the workers met weekly to decide day-to-day matters, while broader issues were to be decided by a management group of workers and patients, which met monthly. However, the doctors who held the contract with the Family Practitioner Com-mittee (see page 116) were legally responsible for everything which went on at the practice, and were, in reality, the employers of the rest of the group. Another important inequality among the work-ers was that we doctors (and other professionals such as the acupuncturist) could supplement our wages with highly-paid part-time work outside; we also gained prestige and approval from feminists and socialists for our commitment in working for a 'low' wage, while the receptionists took home only their wages and received no acclaim for their commitment.

What did we gain from our experience of working there? It was exciting to work in a setting for which we all took responsibility, and which we could change as our ideas and understanding developed. What we both valued most (and now miss) was the support and criticism of a group of people who shared broadly similar values and aims. We did not waste energy swimming against the professional tide, and could reclaim important parts of ourselves which our training had devalued and suppressed, for example humour and spontaneity. The democratic atmosphere allowed us to develop an open, informal approach to staff and patients, which we have been able to bring to our subsequent jobs. We also felt free to be honest with patients and other workers about the stresses affecting our behaviour on a particular day, such as feeling unwell, having a sick child at home, or running late, rather than having to try to appear infallible.

In the workers' group at its best, we were able to share our skills and experiences in a way which is impossible when everybody has a rôle and sticks to it. We learned a lot from working with alternative practitioners – we did not acquire any specific new skills, but their approach taught us to look at people's health problems with a broader perspective than that covered by our training as doctors.

We also learned to help patients gain more control in outside situations, by involving them in decisions about their own health care, and by providing as much information as possible. Even when medical information is made available to people, it may be in incomprehensible jargon, and we learned to fulfil a valuable role as interpreters of such medical mystification. This also applied to patients' records, which are usually kept secret from them. Legally, NHS records are the property of the Secretary of State for Social Services, and it is only convention which stops doctors showing them to patients. In the collective practice, anyone who wanted to could look at their own records, which are a collection of GPs notes, letters from hospitals and others, and results of medical tests. We soon learned that it was necessary to do this with someone nearby to provide explanation and support, as the material may be distressing or insulting – though it is sometimes just disappointingly inadequate. In our subsequent jobs, we have both continued to offer people the opportunity to look at their medical records.

The collective practice developed other important innovations – for example, both the antenatal clinic and the well baby clinic were held in a group setting, with the midwife, health visitors and doctor taking a less controlling role than usual. This allowed women to learn from each other's experience and support each other. The explicit politics of the collective also allowed it to create an atmosphere where women felt safe to reveal things which they might have been reluctant to expose in a conventional practice. Lesbians, for example, knew that their sexuality could be discussed, when relevant, without being focused on as pathological or problematic. Women who had been raped were able to come to us knowing that we would offer sensitive and sympathetic help as well as medical advice and treatment. When women trusted us in these sensitive personal areas, we had to be careful to consult them about what they wanted us to reveal about them if we referred them elsewhere, although we could not ensure that they received equally sympathetic treatment from other agencies.

We do not wish to make a final overall judgement on the practice. Its history demonstrates that no-one can set up a feminist utopia in a single practice; at a time when the very existence of the NHS is under serious threat, we may be forced to use our limited energy to defend it, rather than to develop new structures. But we are proud to have worked in this radical project which for a few years acted as a focus of inspiration for people struggling to find a better way of doing things.

Working within existing structures

Both of us now work in ordinary health centre practices – to what extent have we simply 'sold out' to the liberal general practice establishment? We have already mentioned that our experience in the collective practice helped us to develop a more personal approach to patients and fellow-workers, and that we learned to act as mediators between patients and 'the system', and as communicators of medical information. Working within the existing structure does not mean limiting ourselves to individual relationships with patients. We can, for example, be involved in setting up or supporting groups of women with shared problems, such as the successful menopause group at the health centre where one of us works. Unfortunately, this group also illustrates a major drawback of working within existing structures, namely that other people can limit worthwhile projects: the menopause group is hardly publicised within the building, because the other GPs worry that 'their' patients might receive medical advice which they disagree with.

Working in our health centres would be more fruitful if there were other feminists working with us; we get a lot of warm support from both patients and staff, but almost nothing in the way of constructive, sisterly criticism and feedback like that we received at the collective practice. And if there were other feminists at the health centre, we might be able to work together to challenge some of the established systems of which we feel critical.

In the context of working within the Establishment, perhaps we should seek representation in the influential decision-making organisations in the medical profession, such as the British Medical Association, General Medical Council and Local Medical Committees. Feminists should have a voice in these powerful bodies, and we greatly admire the few feminist doctors who are brave enough to sit on them and face the isolation, frustration, anger and boredom.

We feel it is important, especially in the present political climate, for feminist doctors to be involved in activities which defend the National Health Service. This is not the place for a detailed discussion of the issues involved in defending a system of which we are also very critical. Doctors' support is, however, much valued in campaigns against hospital closures and privatisation of ancillary services. We also need to find effective political ways of expressing our opposition to private medical practice. Patients sometimes ask us to refer them privately to specialists, and it is hard for us to refuse someone with whom we have a good relationship. A few doctors' refusals to refer individuals for private treatment will have little overall impact on the system. And in some areas, such as psychotherapy and abortion provision, we cannot avoid using private practice to supplement the inadequacies of the NHS (see Rakusen 1982).

The Medical Practitioners' Union, which attracts many left-wing doctors, is an organisation where feminists can have a voice and which gives us a base in the trades union movement, but unfortunately it has little real influence, especially under a Conservative government.

Women in Medicine is an organisation of women doctors, medical students and other interested women. It varies in strength in different parts of the country; in some areas its local groups provide a good forum for discussion and a structure for mutual support. It also holds national conferences, publishes a newsletter and stimulates research, for example on the employment and working conditions of women doctors (eg. Schofield & Ward 1985). Doctors for a Woman's Choice on Abortion provides medical influence and backing for the feminist campaigns on women's reproductive rights.

Even within the most conventional structure, general practice offers a unique opportunity to become involved in, influence and be influenced by the lives of a huge variety of women. As doctors we have access to considerable resources, and it is a challenge to learn to use them in a principled, feminist way.

Keeping ourselves sane

Whilst writing this, we have both been aware of how far what we do at work each day falls short of the ideals we have been describing. This is partly because general practice is, by anyone's standards, a stressful job. Although we do not spend our days, as is popularly imagined, making life-or-death decisions, there are other stresses: long, antisocial hours including not only nights and weekends on call, but split shifts with morning and evening surgeries, close contact with many distressed and vulnerable people in a short space of time, and a pressurised workload determined by unpredictable demand.

For feminists, and indeed for socialists, there is the additional stress of trying to work in a politically principled way within a health service and a society which does not share our principles. We are working 'in and against the State' (London–Edinburgh Weekend Return Group 1980). We juggle with our power and professionalism on the one hand and our sisterhood and humanity on the other, patch up the casualties of the system and send them back, we hope, fighting and strengthened. To continue functioning, we know we must set limits to the amount of work we take on and find space and support for ourselves. Or are we indeed 'superwomen' and not like other women we lecture (counsel?) about taking space and finding support for themselves?

On a practical level, we need to sort out our conditions of work in order to survive, and this really means our long, anti-social hours.

> We are well paid – I often wish I could swap money for time.

Nights and weekends on call can be exhausting and make us quite unfit to respond sensitively to anyone after a busy, sleepless night, as well as interfering with the rest of our lives.

> Last night, I spent the 2 hours between 3 and 5 am at the home of an elderly woman and her husband, who was dying of stomach cancer. The night nurses from the district nursing service were there too, and I felt a sense of satisfaction at the care the couple were receiving, and the way they were able to communicate honestly with each other. But when I came home I could not sleep, reflecting on the implications of her remark, 'You know, I think he wants me to go with him. We did everything together'. This morning I groped my way through surgery like a zombie.

Apart from our personal need for time off, which we owe both to ourselves and to those we are close to, we know that we work less well without it. This is not just because we are tired, but because it is easy to become immersed in being a doctor and lose all sense of anyone else's reality, if being a doctor is all that we do. We also get to feel that the long hours and heavy responsibilities justify our privileges, but self-sacrifice is not a political position, and altruism usually covers less admirable motives. For example, we are both susceptible to the thrill of becoming 'indispensable' to our patients, although as feminists we know that it is counter-productive and harmful to make people dependent on us.

We should not confuse dependence with the need for a continuing relationship with our patients. When people call on their GP, they want to see someone whom they know and who knows them. Lack of continuity of care is a major criticism of the NHS, and the recent attempt to limit the use of deputising doctors reflected widespread concern about this issue. Our need for time to ourselves has to be considered within this context.

GPs traditionally get a lot of support from their wives – in fact, the view of general practice we both received as medical students made it difficult to see how one could be a GP without one. Life as a GP is very much easier if we have friends, companions, lovers or spouses with whom we can share the stresses of the day.

Meetings with other GPs may be another way of finding support, but we both find we often feel like outsiders amongst them, and this may be as true amongst women doctors as men. Also, discussions among doctors are usually more competitive than co-operative, and we may come away feeling our confidence undermined rather than strengthened.

As feminists, we seek support in a group of women in similar situations, but should this be just doctors or a more general health workers' group? The workers' group at our collective practice, women's health groups and individual feminists concerned with health care have all provided us with enormous support, stimulation and criticism – but it seems to us that only a limited amount of their energy can be spared to support doctors.

Is it more appropriate, then, to look for support in a group of feminist GPs, if we are lucky enough to work in an area with more than two or three? If this is our only support group, we are likely to lose some of our radical perspective and even degenerate into self-justification and self-pity, forgetting that being at the top of a hierarchy warps one's view of the world. On the other hand, such a group is a much easier setting to look at our feelings about the problems and contradictions we face as GPs.

> I have never forgotten the response of one of the two men at a practice collective workers' meeting, when I was talking about how trapped and uncomfortable I feel about my power as a doctor: He said 'You sound like a man talking about male power.' It is a useful, if painful comparison. We need support but we need to be kept on our toes – we have to be in contact with other feminists, health workers or not, as well as other feminist doctors.

Perhaps the basis of staying sane is to remain realistic in our expectations of ourselves. Providing a service to a huge range of people in our unequal and unfair society is bound to be a juggling act and we are not going to be able to change the world from our surgery chair, nor can we get it right every time. Often there is no right answer, and we cannot be perfect feminists at work, any more than in the rest of our lives – to expect that we could is not only unrealistic but will leave us disillusioned and exhausted.

As Mary Howell emphasises (Howell 1979), 'feminism is real only insofar as we can represent its perspective in the dailiness of our lives.' Our greatest satisfaction as GPs lies within our everyday relationships with individual patients: it is here that our feminism is both most useful and most problematic, as we will discuss in the next section.

WORKING WITH PEOPLE WHO CONSULT US

Most of this section is about feelings and their social and political setting – not only because these are the areas in which feminism had made the greatest contribution, but because they are always central to any GP's work.

Relationships with patients: some general problems

We would like to see our relationship with the women who consult us as that of 'skilled but sisterly helpers' (Leeson & Gray 1978) and we feel most comfortable if we can work in an egalitarian way. But it is very important to remember that, like it or not, we are in a position of authority over people who come to us for medical help. We have the genuine authority which comes from the skill and experience we have been lucky enough to acquire. . . and a great deal of false authority which comes from the inappropriate power we are given by society. Sometimes we can turn this to the patient's advantage: 'I suggest you rest in bed for 48 hours to give your body a chance to get rid of this 'flu virus. I know that'll be hard, but tell your husband and sons that they've got to do the housework, and that's doctor's orders!' (The problem is that we do not have quite enough authority: she may be allowed to take to her bed, but the cleaning, washing and shopping will be there to do when she gets up.)

Our distaste for our position of authority may lead us to pretend it does not exist. Not only does this put relationships between us and the people who consult us on a dishonest footing, but it is also a way of belittling our own achievements and usefulness, as women so often do. Another danger is that if our own authority is not openly acknowledged, we end up expressing it indirectly, and much more dangerously, when under stress – we may become resentful about our long working hours or heavy responsibilities, or suddenly start throwing our weight around when challenged. This is quite an uncomfortable area because it conflicts with our view of ourselves as feminists, but we have noticed that increasing experience and confidence help us to feel easier about acknowledging and using our authority in our work.

Finding a working style which is 'sisterly' but does not deny our authority is linked with another source of difficulty for feminist doctors: coming to terms with public expectations of us. We need to evolve a style which we can adapt to all our patients – of whatever age, sex, race and class. We must each find an approach (including dress, language, etc.) which is comfortable for us and which reflects ourselves – but it must also be broadly acceptable to a wide variety of people, most of whom are not feminists. Of course, once they come to know and trust us, our language and appearance become less important, and fewer eyebrows are raised when we turn up in trousers.

It is easy to underestimate how much doctors' authority and patients' expectations colour both parties' view of what is happening between us:

> On several occasions I have spent some time in what I thought was 'non-directive counselling', enabling a patient to clarify her own needs and work out what course of action was best for her, but at our next meeting she has said 'Thank you for your advice, doctor, I went home and did exactly what you said'.

There is a third dimension to the problem of 'authority'. We must be aware that, as doctors, we are invested with the official authority of the State: in fact, GPs are increasingly called upon to act as agents of the State. We do this each time we write a prescription or a sickness certificate, but we are the key to many other services and benefits such as 'Disabled Driver' badges, supplementary DHSS payments for special diets or extra heating, and re-housing on 'health grounds'. In many areas it is almost impossible for council tenants to be rehoused without a doctor's letter to say that they suffer from an illness which is caused or made worse by their present accommodation. The accommodation in question may be a damp, crumbling, noisy, vandalised slum which would be unsuitable for anyone, regardless of their state of health. But we cannot refuse to participate without penalising the people who seek our help. We can also be involved in forcible admissions to mental hospitals, in taking children from their parents and putting them into care, and in sending elderly people away to old people's homes. Whatever our personal beliefs, and whether we use it or not, we have the power to make those recommendations, which represent a real threat to people.

Women have no reason to trust us, except on the strength of whatever relationship we build between us; our inevitable race and class assumptions as white professional women, and our ageism which makes us insensitive to the needs and feelings of both the young and the elderly, may lead to further mistrust.

If our relationships with patients go wrong, it may be because of what we represent, because of who we are, or because we simply do not get on as individuals. If we do not understand this, we can be surprised and hurt when people seem not to trust us despite our warmly informal manner, our good intentions and our real concern for their well-being. An awareness of the real power relationship helps us to look critically at what we are doing, and to realise that we have to earn people's trust and respect, not expect them as a right. Our training did not prepare us to deal with any of these issues.

Being locked into our authority as doctors is linked with an attitude of professional detachment which can lead to arrogance and insensitivity to people's feelings. Reacting against this, we can try to minimise the barriers between ourselves and the people who come to us for medical help, and to build a relationship like a friendship. But in doing this we make ourselves vulnerable and risk taking on board all the deep distress we encounter every day. This can be exhausting. Building a useful and sisterly relationship involves finding a balance between these two extremes at a level which suits our own style: a certain amount of self-revelation ('I'm sorry I'm not being very attentive this morning, I was up half the night') can be very helpful, both in reminding the patient that the doctor is human too, and in making the most of our energy to provide a good service. ('Perhaps you could make a double appointment at the end of the week: I'll be more helpful then'.)

'A woman's right to choose'

It is apt that 'a woman's right to choose' is probably the best-known feminist slogan, because choice is exactly what most women are deprived of – not only choice about abortion, but about every facet of our lives. Few women have economic independence and, without this, the majority have few choices, but powerlessness can also make it difficult to see those choices they do have. Pointing these out and encouraging women to use them for their own well-being and happiness is a major part of our work.

These choices may be on a practical level – for example, in the collective practice we were able to offer women the choice of various conventional and alternative treatments. Most of the time, though, we are encouraging women to look at choices which affect them much more intimately. This is not as straightforward as it may sound. We are critical when other doctors impose their world-view on people's lives – for example, labelling women who wish to continue paid work as uncaring mothers – but our feminist principles are also a world-view. Imposing this is not only doomed to failure, but would achieve nothing in terms of the woman's self-esteem and confidence – we would be using our power to determine what is right for the woman, rather than encouraging her to decide. The other extreme would be to support all women uncritically, no matter what choice they made, thereby denying our experience as women, feminists and doctors, as well as denying our power.

We are constantly trying to maintain a balance between inflexible dogmatism and uncritical support – a common example of this is deciding how we can help a woman who lives with a violent man and 'chooses' to remain. She carries a double burden of guilt – that she has somehow caused or even deserves the violence she suffers and also that she does not have the strength to leave. Her friends and family tell her, and she may even agree, that she is a fool to stay, but male violence to women is largely condoned in our society, and we internalise the prevailing view that 'she must have deserved it'. Meanwhile the radio plays 'Stand by your man'. If she leaves she must not only break her emotional ties and perhaps face extreme violence, but also negotiate a hostile system in an attempt to find money and accommodation. Her choice can only be made from a very small range of options and if we ignore this, we may leave her paralysed by feelings of guilt; on the other hand, if we support her uncritically within the situation, we may allow her to tolerate it longer than she would otherwise have done.

Similar conflicts arise when adolescents come to us asking for contraception. We support their 'right to a self-determined sexuality' (one of the demands of the Women's Liberation Movement) but often their sexuality is largely dictated by outside forces – the media, the fear of being left out, pressure from boys, and so on. Sometimes we cannot bring ourselves to ask young women about their sexual enjoyment – at least two-thirds of them say 'well, he seems to like it'. Not only are they not enjoying sex, but they seem to have no expectation that they might. Of course, we are willing to provide contraception, but we also want to find a way of helping them find our what they want from sex and life. Yet the same forces that push young women into sexual relationships which they may not want also characterise adults as killjoys who want to stop young people having fun. We find our status as powerful adults makes it almost impossible to talk about these issues with young women without being seen as authoritarian, which prevents any two-way discussion. During the time that we were writing this, it became illegal for us to advise anyone under 16 about contraception without their parents' consent. We welcomed the House of Lords ruling which reversed this change in the law, which had begun to have disastrous effects on the well-being of young women and made it very much harder for us to develop helpful relationships with them.

Young women often see their mothers as authoritarian and restrictive, and we become involved in this too because, as the mother's GP, we may be asked for help and support with her fears about the situation. Usually her concern is chiefly with protecting her daughter from early motherhood and shotgun marriage – she may have experienced this herself and know how hard it can be. We cannot forget that we are family doctors working in a community, whatever our criticisms of the family or community as institutions may be. We need to support both the adolescent women and their mothers and try to reconcile the apparent and real conflicts of interest, respecting medical confidentiality and our interlocking relationships. Similar and even more difficult situations may arise when we act as confidante and supporter to two or more women involved with the same man (who, in general, does not come to see us at all, of course).

A woman's right to choose may also mean a woman making a choice which we see as a bad one for her.

> I remember one woman in particular, whom I referred for an abortion. I knew her well, and was convinced that an abortion would be disastrous for her. In this case, as in others, I had misjudged the situation, but I find it difficult if it turns out that a woman's choice has disastrous consequences that I have foreseen. Ideally, I support her through her distress while helping her to understand what has happened without blaming herself. In practice, I often have to wrestle with my feelings of resentment at her 'stupidity', although I know these feelings are unfair.

Sometimes the greatest struggle is to allow a woman the choice not to discuss things with us. She may come to us for a service – referral to another agency, a sick note because she is too distressed to work – but she is handling the situation herself and does not want us to be involved. Our training as caring GPs urges us to probe deeper, but this may be an intrusion. If, for example, a woman has come to a firm decision that she needs an abortion, do we have a right to involve ourselves beyond ensuring that this is medically possible and is really what she wants?

Many choices we may wish to offer women involve us in extra work – home births are the major example of this. We need to be available 24 hours a day for a month – two weeks before and after the date on which the baby is due – and then be prepared to leave whatever we are doing once labour is under way. This can be very disruptive, not only of our own lives (one of the few days we had together working on this chapter was taken over by a home birth) but also of those of our other patients. Home deliveries, although stressful and demanding, can also be very rewarding and we develop very special relationships with women who request them. Similarly, it is easy to work closely and rewardingly with women who share our world-view. It is tempting to devote a lot of our time and energy to these women, but if we do, this is at the expense of women less like ourselves with whom we feel less empathy. This is much the same as the tendency of doctors in general to favour articulate middle-class patients.

Don't blame the victim

The recognition that individual women can, and often wish to, take responsibility for their own lives, does not alter the fact that most of the factors causing disease are beyond our individual control: for example, poverty, poor housing and work conditions, unemployment, pollution. But a lot of today's preventive medicine and health education emphasise individuals' responsibility for their own ill-health, and blame the victims rather than the social pressures which make them unhealthy. Women, in particular, come in for a good deal of blame: not only for their own problems but those of their children, husbands and parents.

Smokers, people who over-eat, people who escape from their problems with tranquillisers or alcohol – all end up with an overwhelming feeling of personal guilt, which is useless as well as uncomfortable. Undermining people's self-esteem does not help them to change their unhealthy behaviour.

How can a feminist approach help us? Ideally, we need to strive to understand the pressures which bring about a woman's unhealthy behaviour, both in the particular circumstances of her own life and in our society in general, for example, the pervasive images of idealised women's bodies in advertising. Then perhaps we can share our analysis with the patient herself, and work out a plan of action together, so that she can take more control over her own health. This involves both of us understanding the many factors which make this difficult for her. In other words, the doctor becomes an ally helping the woman take control, rather than being yet another outside pressure on her.

These ideas are very hard to put into practice in a ten-minute appointment. Not all women will accept this approach, and we are often faced with the problem of how we relate to women who want treatment which as doctors we see as useless and harmful, and which as feminists we see as a damaging response to sexual stereotypes. Slimming pills are a particular bogey for both of us: they do not work in the long term, have unpleasant side-effects and may be addictive. They also hold out to women the hope of a magic, individual solution to what is essentially a political problem: the unreal images to which women are expected to conform. When a woman tells us that her marriage will break up if she does not lose weight, that this is her last chance, that she has tried every known diet, Weight Watchers and a compulsive eating group, that she understands the risks of slimming pills and still thinks it worth it... are we justified in using our authority to with-hold them? Slimming pills are no more harmful than dozens of other widely-used drugs, for many of which there is no real proof of long-term effectiveness (eg. Valium). And the other side of this society's slimness fetish is the punitive attitude it (and its doctors) take towards obesity. Will she be able to differentiate our principled position from the punitive attitude of her previous doctor who belittled the problem, stressed will-power, implied that she was greedy or self-indulgent and totally failed to respond to her distress? How do we respond to her distress and avoid adding to her guilt and low self-esteem, without going along with her analysis and accepting her solution? We often fail.

> At one recent morning surgery, one woman left in tears and another vowed to change doctors, because I refused them slimming pills.

On the other hand, the occasional 'success' makes the feminist approach seem worthwhile. Women who over-eat often do so in response to needs other than hunger (Orbach 1978; 1982); frequently it is for comfort, or to suppress anger.

> Sometimes I ask a patient to write down not only everything she eats, but also what she feels at the time. The most striking example I can remember is 'I had a row with my daughter when she came home at midnight, and then ate a quart of icecream from the freezer.' Discussing what she has written, we can develop an understanding of what her eating habits mean for her, and then find a way of changing it... or sometimes the focus of the consultation shifts from the food to the feelings themselves and other ways of dealing with them.

Difficult issues of guilt, blame and responsibility also arise when women come in with family problems, either with children who, for example, do not sleep or refuse to go to school, or with marital problems. It is not unusual for a couple to come together to see us and present the woman as 'ill' because she is bad-tempered and resentful, or because she no longer responds sexually. Very often there is almost a collusion between the husband, who appears very caring and concerned, and the wife, to lay all the blame on her and deny that he has any responsibility. They wish to find a physical basis for the problem, preferably one which can be treated with pills. The recent publicity given to premenstrual tension is a very mixed blessing, as it can be used to explain away women's bursts of anger about real sources of dissatisfaction in their lives. Our response to these situations often involves a compromise. Our analysis stems from our commitment to women's well-being, informed by our own feminist perspective, but we have to recognise that the couple do not share our world-view and may not be interested in making far-reaching, uncomfortable changes in their attitudes and lives.

The sisterhood in women's lives

When women find a sympathetic woman doctor who is prepared to listen, they often unburden themselves, perhaps for the first time, of painful personal problems. It is very easy for these women to become dependent on the doctor. This is rather gratifying for us, but results in the woman having less control over her life. One important way of avoiding this is to encourage women to find sisterly support outside the surgery. This means asking them about friends, sisters, mothers, daughters in whom they might or do confide. This is an easy and accessible idea ('a trouble shared is a trouble halved') rather than a piece of high-flown psychotherapy. Some women may find it hard to expose themselves in this way, though, and sometimes the family may not be an appropriate place for a woman to seek support because of her existing role within it.

It is also possible to put women in touch with groups set up by women with particular shared difficulties and interests – for example, a menopause group which is part of the local women's health group and a mastectomy support group at our local hospital. Referrals to compulsive eating groups, Women's Aid, Rape Crisis Centres or other feminist agencies may also be useful. It can be very helpful to put individuals with a shared difficulty in touch with each other, although we must be scrupulous about seeking permission first. For example, one of us introduced two pregnant nineteen-year-olds, who each felt too shy to go to antenatal classes alone.

Nevertheless, sometimes the doctor really is the only person the woman feels able to confide in. We may be able to do nothing and have no useful advice to offer, but just being there as a listening ear is genuinely healing. It is a delicate and unequal relationship, and one problem is how much the doctor should say about herself and her own experiences. It is not hard for us to talk about our own experiences of having coils fitted, self-help remedies for cystitis or Maureen's children's love of junk food, but we are both more reticent about our personal relationships. We must remember that the time women spend with their GP may be the only space they get to themselves and we could easily crowd them out if we are too intrusive. Also, we have to remember that what a patient tells us is protected by medical confidentiality, but what we tell her is not. People enjoy discussing their doctors and in both the communities in which we work, gossip travels very fast.

Another pitfall is that the sharing of our experience as women with patients may make them feel that they are not as good at fulfilling a woman's role as we are.

> Many women know that I have two small children and some know that I do not live with their father. They often seem impressed that, in this situation, I also manage a demanding job, and see me as some kind of superwoman. I feel a fraud, because they do not know how disorganised my life really is, despite my many advantages compared with most single mothers. Although I am gratified by their admiration, the competitive atmosphere between us upsets me. Recently a woman who was half an hour late for a 10.15 appointment explained that this was because of the difficulty of getting out with two small children. I was relieved that I stopped myself (although only just) from saying 'I have two small children and I'm here by 9 o'clock'.

Helping women to get what they need

Many women's lives are dominated by the constant outpouring of emotional and practical support in their role as carers. This is most obvious within a family, where women in their 50s may find themselves caring for elderly relatives and neighbours, a husband, children and grandchildren. It also happens in most situations shared by men and women – work, friendships, clubs. These demands may overlap and the woman may become pig-in-the-middle – a phrase many of them have used to us. Women act as emotional safety valves. They absorb the tensions and problems, and provide support for everyone. With no-one to do the same for them, they may develop physical and emotional manifestations of stress. This role is largely unrecognised and always devalued. It is taken for granted, often even by the woman herself, as a natural attribute of women.

> This was brought home to one woman when her husband had a heart attack. She not only supported him emotionally, spending hours at his bedside, but also took on all the practical and financial problems and continued her own job. She was simultaneously supporting her daughter through a marriage break-up. A few weeks later she took an accidental overdose of tranquillisers. Her husband, although he knew she had taken too many pills, left her in a deep sleep for 36 hours before calling a doctor. When she came to see me the

next week, she poured out her enormous anger and hurt that a man for whom she had so recently done so much could be so selfish and callous. She realised he had become self-centred over the years and particularly since his illness. She went home and confronted him – forcing him to recognise, and claiming for herself, her strength, energy and commitment.

Women may feel they have no right to ask for time and space for themselves, although lack of these is often the main problem underlying the symptoms which bring them to the doctor. They come instead on the pretext of some minor physical, and therefore respectable, complaint, or of seeking help for someone else – usually a child or husband. Even when the woman has found a space to express her distress, she may still feel guilty about it. As many as half of the women who have unburdened themselves to us say as they leave 'I'm sorry to have wasted your time' – not only feeling that their distress is unimportant, but also devaluing what has passed between us.

This feeling of having no right to her own space is not limited to the medical field. It often permeates a woman's whole life, making it generally bleak and unsatisfying as well as undermining her health. She lacks 'True Rest' – this term, which originates from the Pellin Centre, means some activity which restores a person's strength and sense of well-being. Examples of traditional ways in which men find True Rest are angling and football. Sometimes when we ask women how they would spend their time for themselves if they had any, they are unable to think of anything. Sometimes it is sitting and knitting – usually for other people!

> I like to 'prescribe' True Rest on a prescription form – writing 'one hour's reading, three times a week', for example. As well as ensuring that my suggestion is not forgotten under the pressure of shopping, work, collecting the children, helping the neighbours, etc., the prescription often provides a useful talking point for the rest of the family and is an appropriate substitute for the expected tranquillisers.

The low self-esteem of women often comes up in consultations. We have learnt through feminism how women undervalue their real achievements of, for example, bringing up a family, because society in general undervalues them. We cannot help women to value themselves unless we value them. Women also often lack sources of feelings of accomplishment in their lives, and sometimes it is possible, even in a short consultation, to help a woman find more purpose for herself, as Maureen's GP did for her as a child.

Recently I talked to a woman who asked for help because she felt unenthusiastic about sex with her husband. I said 'Tell me a little about the rest of your life'. She described a sense of frustration and boredom with her life as a housewife and mother of two small children aged 2 and 4, with a part-time 'little' job. She did not feel overtired, was very fond of her husband and did not dislike housework, childcare, or her 'little' job – but she felt that she wanted more. We talked about possibilities and she decided to apply for a part-time secretarial course. Next time I saw her she had recovered her enthusiasm for life in general. I am not sure whether her sexual feelings had changed, but this no longer seemed to be a problem.

The most consciously authoritarian technique I (occasionally) use is to set 'homework' for patients, and sometimes the hardest task is to persuade them to do something to please themselves. A woman who easily found time to keep a conscientious weekly diary of her eating habits, mostly because she felt it would please me, took about ten weeks to buy a small bunch of flowers for herself.

Working with male patients

Working with male patients can be difficult for a feminist, but can also provide unique opportunities for bringing some of the insights of feminism to men. As most men have a woman in their life from whom they get emotional support, we are less likely to see men complaining of emotional stress, although they often come with anxiety-related problems. When men do bring emotional problems, they often choose a woman doctor – presumably because they prefer a woman to fulfil the womanly role of listening ear. We also often already know the man from the account of a woman who is close to him before actually meeting him; this reverses the common situation of a woman being defined by her relationship to a man. These factors often mean we are in a position to put forward to men a more woman-centred way of looking at the world.

It is not easy to find a way to help a man who confesses to beating up his wife, an unemployed man who feels unmanly and resentful because his wife is the breadwinner, and cannot bring himself to do any housework while she is out at work, or a man who complains of sexual difficulties but insists on viewing these as a mechanical problem unrelated to feelings or relationships. We do not want to fall into the trap of being 'understanding' and not questioning their assumptions about male rights. On the other hand, as with all the patients we find it hard to deal with, we have a responsibility to provide continuing medical care, and we can neither make every consultation into an ideological battle, nor choose not to relate to them. Some men might solve the problem by choosing to see a male doctor, but they do not all do so, so we have to find ways of meeting their challenge.

Sometimes there are rewarding encounters with men who are prepared to discuss their role and their feelings openly with us.

> Recently I saw a 44-year-old man who said 'I just don't feel right. Is it the male menopause?' He then told me that his children, aged 17 and 21, were becoming independent and would soon leave home. He respected their independence, but was sad to realise that he would soon lose his rewarding role as a father. We talked about other ways he could find purpose and satisfaction in the second half of his life.

Some men feel as burdened as women by the conventional expectations of their role.

> A 61-year-old man came to see me complaining of weight loss; after tests to exclude physical illnesses, and some discussion, it became clear that he was very depressed because he was made redundant last year. I was not surprised that he felt very anxious about his greatly reduced income, or that he found his days empty and unfulfilling; the main source of his depressed feelings, however, was guilt that he is unable to provide for his wife as he was brought up to do.

In such situations, seeing a doctor who questions society's assumptions about male and female roles may help a man to feel less guilty and inadequate, and to find strength and a broader perspective with which to face the real, painful problems of unemployment.

Unfortunately, we are often unable to avoid reinforcing sex roles, which tend to become more rigid under stress such as physical illness when it may not seem an appropriate time to challenge them. For example, when a man needs to modify his diet, it is usually necessary to discuss this with his wife if there is to be any chance of change. We are thus confirming her in the role of unpaid cook and dietician. But we can at least comment on what is happening, even if we cannot change it.

CONCLUSION

We hope that this chapter has given some idea of what we mean by a feminist approach to general practice. It is a patchwork of the personal, the political and the pragmatic. The contradictions of our position lead to constant compromises: how much we compromise, and which compromises we choose to make, will vary at different stages in our own lives, as well as varying between individuals according to our differing experiences and personalities, and the places and situations we find ourselves in. We can use a feminist perspective to increase our understanding of women's health needs and of our own position; we can find ways of sharing skills and knowledge with other women; we can be involved in campaigning on women's health issues; we can attempt, if we are brave, to fight the sexism of the medical profession and the health care system; we can try to set up alternative feminist structures.

Above all, we can try to carry out our own daily work in a principled, feminist way. This includes just being a good doctor! Our emphasis on the psychological, social and political side of our work may have obscured the fact that we spend a lot of our time dealing with people who are ill. There is no point in endlessly analysing the contradictions of our position if we do not remember to treat people with respect, to be aware of their embarrassment and fear, to take care to explain what we are doing and give information about the drugs we prescribe, and to warm our hands and instruments before examining someone.

We are sometimes asked why we continue to practise orthodox medicine when we are critical about its content as well as about its hierarchical structure. The heart of the matter for us both is the opportunity it gives us to be involved with almost everyone in our community: 90 per cent of people visit their GP in a five-year period. In a way nothing could bring us closer to women's lives, and that is the true privilege which we value most.

Acknowledgements

Many thanks to Lucy Tinkler who typed the manuscript, to Kathy Levine who took care of Maureen's children while we were writing, and to the friends who read and commented on our first draft, especially Shirley Read, Annabel Page, Sophie Laws and Maggie Helliwell.

We would also like to thank some of the many people who have helped us to develop as doctors and to evolve a feminist approach to our work: Maggie's mother, Dr. Gisela Eisner, and Maureen's first GP, Dr. Keith Wood; Anna Farrow and Peter Fleming of the Pellin Centre; the Essex Road (Islington) Women's Health Group of 1975–1976; all our fellow-workers at the Limes Grove Practice from 1977–1982; and, most important of all, the women who have consulted us as patients.

Useful Addresses

Doctors for a Woman's Choice on Abortion: 101 Burbage Road, London SE 24
Medical Practitioners' Union: 79 Camden Road, London NW1 9ES
Pellin Centre: 43 Killyon Road, London SW8 2XS
Pelling Training Courses: 15 Killyon Road, London SW8 2XS
Politics of Health Group: c/o BSSRS, 9 Poland Street, London W1
Women in Medicine: 34 Hunter House Road, Sheffield 11
Women's Health Information Centre: 52 Featherstone Street, London EC 1

References and Further Reading

Anderson A & McPherson A ed (1983) *Women's Problems in General Practice*. Oxford University Press
Berger J & Mohr J (1976) *A Fortunate Man*. London: Writers' and Readers' Publishing Cooperative
The CATCALL Collective eds (1983) Feminist Politics and Women's Health Special Issue. *Catcall*, **15**, 1–25 (obtainable from 37 Wortley Road, London E 6)
The CATCALL Collective eds (1984) Feminist Politics and Women's Health Special Issue. *Catcall*, **16**, 2–31
Chamberlain M (1981) *Old Wives' Tales*. London: Virago
Cooke M & Ronalds C (1985) Women doctors in urban general practice: the patients. *British Medical Journal*, **290**, 753–755
Cooke M & Ronalds C (1985) Women doctors in urban general practice: the doctors. *British Medical Journal*, **290**, 755–758
Day P (1982) *Women Doctors: Choice and Constraints for Medical Manpower*. London: King's Fund Centre (obtainable from 126 Albert Street, London NW1 7NA)
Doyal L (1979) *The Political Economy of Health*. London: Pluto Press
Ehrenreich B & English D (1979) *For Her Own Good: 150 Years of the Experts' Advice to Women*. London: Pluto Press
Howell M (1979) Can we be feminists and professionals? *Women's Studies International Quarterly*, **2**, 1–7 (published by Pergamon Press)
Leeson J & Gray J (1978) *Women and Medicine*. London: Tavistock
London–Edinburgh Weekend Return Group ed (1980) *In and Against the State*. London: Pluto Press
Mitchell J (1984) *What is to be done about Illness and Health?* Harmondsworth: Penguin
Orbach S (1978) *Fat is a Feminist Issue I*. Feltham: Hamlyn
Orbach S (1982) *Fat is a Feminist Issue II*. Feltham: Hamlyn
Rakusen J (1982) Feminism and the politics of health. *Medicine in Society*, **8**, 17–25 (obtainable from 16 St John Street, London EC 1)

Roberts H ed (1981) *Women, Health and Reproduction.* London: Routledge & Kegan Paul

Saffron L (1985) Clinical smears: problems with well women clinics. *Trouble & Strife,* **5**, 13–17 (obtainable from 50 Bethel Street, Norwich, Norfolk)

Schofield P & Ward G (1985) Women in general practice: provision for maternity leave for general practitioners. *British Medical Journal,* **290**, 525–526

8

Experiences of Counselling Women

MERRYN COOKE

About the Author

I am not sure when I first saw myself as a feminist. Being white and middle class gave me many privileges. I went to a girls' school, had no brothers, and my parents encouraged me to have a career, to travel and to be independent. I went to college in Liverpool in the 1960s and became much more aware of class and racist discrimination than of being oppressed myself for being female. I believed I could influence American policy in Vietnam but it never entered my head that I could challenge my GP or say what I wanted in bed!

After leaving University I worked as a teacher for nine years, mainly in Southern Africa, followed by three-and-a-half years as a research assistant in England. I joined a women's group in England in 1974 for a year and again in 1980 when I returned from Africa. It was in these groups, recalling incidences and experiences – often very similar to other women's – and reading books such as The Female Eunuch, Against Our Will *and* Our Bodies, Ourselves *that I saw how I had been living by rules and within limits defined by men. I remembered travelling from college to the Brook Advisory Clinic in Birmingham, the nearest place I could get the pill, and being told by my GP as he gave me Valium that my nerves would improve if I got married. I recalled fears and experiences of sexual violence and how in many relationships I had dressed, talked and acted only to please the men I was with. I was inspired by many women who were actively challenging the patriarchal status quo.*

In 1980 I joined a Rape Crisis Line as a volunteer and from 1983 to 1984 helped at a Well Women's Clinic attached to a general practice, again as a volunteer. I am now 39 years old and enjoying the challenges and rewards of being a student nurse.

When I started working as a volunteer counsellor at the Rape Crisis Line and Well Women's Clinic I had had no formal counselling training. I was aware of my anger and frustration, fears and sadness at how women are oppressed and I wanted to channel these into effecting a change for women, including myself. In the past four years the experience of this work has made me clearer about the ways in which I can be effective in achieving this.

Firstly, I subscribe to the core conditions of client-centred counselling as defined by Carl Rogers. Rogers (1967) describes the relationship between the client and counsellor in which the counsellor must possess empathy, genuineness and a respect for the client's potential to lead her own life and utilise her own resources. I believe I have no right to tell women how to act or feel, but by active listening I hope to enable women to talk in safety without fear of being judged, to express their feelings, to gain a clearer understanding of their problems and to be able to make their own decisions on how to resolve them. Although I can give information, I cannot provide answers to someone else's problems. I am not an 'expert' and I often need help myself.

I need to understand my fears and prejudices that might get in the way of giving full attention to women I hope to help. It has therefore been important to explore my own feelings – for instance about male violence – when working for the Rape Crisis Line.

However, I would not be true to myself or the women I see if I did not challenge many of their negative feelings of guilt and worthlessness. Women so often blame themselves and feel guilty for events over which they have no control. 'Blaming the victim' is a classic way to avoid accepting responsibility for an abuse of power, whether it be men accusing women of 'provoking rape' or doctors defining for all women 'the best way to give birth'. Guilt, fear and ignorance can paralyse women, and it is only when they feel they have the right to better treatment by family, police or health service, when they are confident in their ability to ask or argue for such treatment, and feel secure that others are supporting them in their actions that they can effect change.

In all the counselling I take part in there is an obligation on my part to provide women with as much information as possible before they make choices. This should not be giving directive advice like that on many problem pages by agony aunts and health workers, but discussing with women the 'pros and cons' of possible courses of action or giving factual information, for example on the law of incest or different forms of contraception.

As a feminist, one of the main aims of my work is to help liberate women from roles defined for them by a patriarchal society and to give them a real choice of how they wish to live their lives. I therefore find it impossible to counsel in isolation from political work, and feel that I cannot sit and discuss with a woman the limited options available to her unless I am actively involved in trying to widen those options. In a similar way, giving money to feed starving people might make me feel nice but does not help them to become more self-reliant or challenge the economic and political arrangements that contribute to their poverty.

Finally, it is important for me that the structure within which I work is an expression of the political aims of the workers. Both the Rape Crisis Line and the Well Women's Clinic work as a collective – we believe that all women's feelings are valid, and that by sharing skills and experiences we can learn from each other. We learn to trust each other and build a supportive network for ourselves. As an individual and as part of a group I can then offer women support as they attempt to take control of their lives and health. I have tried to use these ideas in my work in both settings, and I shall describe both kinds of counselling and try to convey how these principles are translated into practice.

RAPE CRISIS LINE

The background

Although women are discriminated against in the economic, legal and educational spheres, many campaigns have been successful in breaking down barriers to women in jobs, training and legal rights. But it is the social and personal roles imposed on women which are the hardest to change. Although men often have economic sanctions over their wives, girlfriends and children they also use physical violence – sanctioned by society – to force women to conform to male-defined sexual and social roles. In many cases, physical and sexual violence are inseparable.

One of the effects of the rise of the women's liberation movement in the late 1960s and 1970s was the open expression of women's anger at the violence they had personally experienced from men, at the way women are degraded and defined in pornography, and at the belittling of women's experience by jokes about rape. Books such as *Against Our Will* by Susan Brownmiller (1977) chronicled the history of male violence and rape.

The first practical response was the setting up of Women's Aid Refuges for women and their children wanting to leave violent partners. Women were demanding that the scale and reality of domestic violence be taken seriously, that it should no longer be socially acceptable for men to beat women, and that the state should provide homes for women rather than accuse them of being 'intentionally homeless'. In the same way, the Rape Crisis Lines which started in England in the 1970s not only offered women the opportunity – often for the first time – to talk about their experiences in a sympathetic environment but, by their existence, demanded that society recognise the appalling reality and consequences of rape or incest. They took the blame away from women and placed it back on men who abuse their positions of power.

When talking to women who have been sexually abused, it is important to understand their fears – fears of not being believed and often of being judged guilty of provoking the assault. The myths surrounding rape are responsible for these fears because, as they are myths, no women's experiences fit the stereotype. Nevertheless, this stereotype is internalised by women and they blame themselves for what has happened.

Myths and realities about rape

The myths are many but include:

> Women want to be dominated and enjoy 'rough' sex.
> Women lead men on, they are provocative and say 'no' when they mean 'yes'.
> If women kept their legs together they couldn't be raped.
> Rapes occur (at night) in dark alleyways.
> Rapists are strangers to the women they assault.
> Most rapes are unplanned – men's sexual urges are too strong and they suddenly lose control.
> The only rapist who plans his attack is mentally ill – a 'sex fiend'.
> Rape is just sex you don't really want.

The reality is very different. Women of all ages, colours and classes are raped, as are physically and mentally disabled women, wives and single women. None I have ever known has enjoyed the experience of sexual assault, be it sexual harrassment at work, being fondled by an uncle, 'flashed' at in the park, or group rape and buggery. Rape is an act of violence whether it is beating, strangling, forcing objects into the anus or vagina or forced intercourse. There is either actual violence or the threat of violence, sometimes more than one man is involved, and verbal abuse is commonplace. Approximately half of all rapists are known to the women they rape, and in the case of child abuse over

90 per cent of abusers are trusted adults. Many rapes take place in the home of the woman or rapist, and not just in parks, offices, cars or trains. The myth that men suddenly lose control is shown to be false by the fact that most rape and child abuse is planned. Men arrange for women to be alone, carry weapons to threaten with or to use, break into homes, or go with other men to overpower a woman. Most rapists are not mentally ill – they are ordinary sons, friends and husbands. Only three per cent of convicted rapists are referred for psychiatric treatment.

Women's experiences rarely fit the stereotype. If a woman reports a rape to the police she may be accused of leading the man on, or of not resisting if she cannot show evidence of bruising or torn clothing. If she knew the man, the woman may lose all trust in her own judgement of people and feel very vulnerable. She may feel degraded and dirty and want to wash compulsively. Some women who suffered long-term abuse as children have very little self-regard and feel they have no rights to have their bodies respected. Women start to blame themselves for 'taking a taxi', 'walking home with him' or 'wearing a short skirt', and these feelings are often reinforced by a judge's pronouncements in court. Women feel guilty for not shouting or struggling, even though they were petrified and being threatened. They are afraid of being in the same situations as when they were raped, and so cannot take taxis, work in the same office or be alone at home. They may fear both reprisals from the rapists if they report them and the reactions of friends, family or lovers, who may suspect that the women were to blame. There is also the natural fear of any future sexual contact or any close contact with men.

Working on a Rape Crisis Line

My work is aimed at allowing women to talk about their experiences and feelings. By believing their story and accepting their distress, I can hopefully help them start to work through the shame, hurt and fear and come to terms with what has happened. By challenging their feelings of self-blame I hope to help them to express anger at the rapist and put the blame on to him. I can also reassure women that they are not alone or unusual in their reactions and that they are not 'mad'. There are no easy cures for the effects of rape, no panacea for the fear that all women know of sexual assault. But we can give moral and some practical support such as help with re-housing for women fearing reprisals, self-defence classes to help women feel more assertive, and contact with groups such as Incest Survivors. We can give information on the law and medical procedures, accompany women to court or the police, arrange for them to see a sympathetic woman doctor, or help them claim Criminal Injuries Compensation.

The most important task is still to be there as often as a woman needs, to listen to her, believe in what she says, and empathise without judgement with what she has to say. It is also essential to support her in whatever she decides to do to regain control, and not to prescribe or judge one way as better than another. Advice to 'Find a nice man to look after you and settle down' ignores the reality of women's feelings after assault and the extent of violence in the home.

Women volunteers at the Rape Crisis Line where I work go through a training course which the group itself runs. There are usually about ten evening meetings and two full days. There are sessions dealing with factual information about matters such as the law and police procedure, but most emphasis is put upon sharing our experiences and ideas about sexual violence. We also talk specifically about sexuality and racism. We need to look at our own sexuality and our prejudices so that we do not fall into the pattern of assuming that all women are heterosexual or wish to be. There have been historical links between rape and racism, especially in relation to American slavery, but it is important that we confront the issue today. The police and courts are more likely to believe white women and more likely to arrest and convict black men, and we need to look at our own racism and work out ways to counsel women who may themselves by overtly racist. At the full day meetings we concentrate on counselling practice and sharing experiences of how we have worked in the past. Our aims are that volunteers and new women can share skills, learn to trust each other and be mutually supportive. I feel this support is vital because we nearly always work in pairs. This is so that women benefit from having two people to relate to and are more likely to find someone to get on with. When we give talks to other organisations or groups we can offer several points of view and different experiences. We also need support for ourselves because much of what we hear is distressing, and it is very stressful to answer the phone alone. When we take it in turns to answer the phone or visit a woman together, there is the opportunity to shout or cry between calls, offer support and praise to the other volunteer, and talk about the calls or visit. Not all Rape Crisis Lines work in this way but I find it very helpful.

Apart from answering the phone, we also talk to women face to face and are happy to talk to relatives, social workers, teachers and others. We meet once a week to discuss policy and administration and talk over any important calls. We try to share tasks such as publicity and finance, though much of this falls on the two part-time paid workers. We are often asked to talk to groups such as Housewives' Register, police trainees or youth clubs. I feel it is important to raise people's awareness of the reality and extent of sexual abuse and so help in pressing for changes in the law and court procedure and in the ways the media report rape. It is also vital to work to increase the number of women police surgeons, and especially to change police attitudes, for I have talked to women who seemed more upset at the treatment they received at the police station than with the actual assault. I feel it is important that society knows the reality of rape so that women and children who have suffered sexual abuse will receive sympathy and support, and this political work is an integral part of my 'counselling' – if it were successful, Rape Crisis Lines would be redundant.

Many of these ways of working are shared with the other counselling setting I shall describe, as are some of the stereotypes about women and their feelings in response.

WELL WOMEN'S CLINIC

In 1983 I was asked by a health visitor attached to a general practice if I would like to help at a Well Women's Clinic which was about to open. I had been involved in running some sessions on women's health courses, and many women there had expressed interest in well women's clinics and voiced their wish to have more time to talk over individual health problems. The health visitor was keen to have some volunteers with counselling experience rather than only formally trained health workers, and I was interested to see how my feminist ideas fitted into a general practice setting.

The background to Well Women's Clinics

In the past decade, as a result of pressure from women workers in the National Health Service, ordinary women dissatisfied with their NHS treatment and feminists in women and health groups, there have been calls for an improvement in health services provided for women and campaigns have been mounted for well women's clinics.

The main points of dissatisfaction expressed by women in the town where I live were:

1 The lack of time available to talk to doctors and other health professionals, which meant that women were only 'allowed' to discuss very specific issues rather than general health problems.

2 The fact that women had little self-confidence to challenge a health worker's decision or ask for more information.

3 An over-emphasis on drug therapy and lack of information about alternative treatments.

4 Too few women doctors, especially in general practice and gynaecology.

There are now a number of Well Women's Clinics in my area but they are very varied. Some are simply cervical cytology and family planning clinics, and some have women doctors, trained health personnel and volunteers working in them. Others are run by volunteers and are more of a resource centre where women can talk to other women about their health. Many offer some form of counselling as well as factual information. The clinic where I worked was unusual in that it was part of a group general practice and access was limited to patients registered with that practice.

Why have a Well Women's Clinic

The practice is located in an inner city area and, of the eight GPs, only one is a woman. The two health visitors and woman doctor felt strongly that local women needed more access to health information and discussion than was possible during a normal surgery consultation and that they should all have the opportunity to see a woman doctor. There was a feeling that many women wanted preventive services and advice for gynaecological or breast problems, but were too embarrassed to ask their male GP. Therefore, the practice decided to start a weekly clinic aiming to:

(*a*) offer health information and advice, including alternatives and complements to conventional medicine;

(*b*) give women an opportunity to talk to other women about their health and to integrate the social, emotional and physical aspects of their lives;

(*c*) share knowledge and skills, and give confidence to women to ask their own GP for help;

(*d*) give patients of the practice a chance to consult a woman doctor who could also offer preventive services such as cervical smears.

The practice doctors agreed to a Well Women's Clinic starting for one year in the first instance.

How the clinic worked

Apart from the health visitors and the female GP, other health workers attached to the practice helped at the clinic, including the midwife and psychiatric social worker. Volunteers included ex-nurses, community workers from the Asian Women's Refuge, nurse tutors and a GP with a special interest in the menopause, and several of the volunteers were patients at the practice.

The clinic opened once a week between 5pm and 7pm. We used five rooms: a consulting room, two small interview rooms, and a playroom for children next to the largest room where we welcomed women, had tea or coffee and displayed books, leaflets and videos. We tried to make the atmosphere as friendly and relaxed as possible, and women were welcomed by one worker, who offered a drink and explained how the clinic was run. All women were given the opportunity to talk in private to one volunteer and could consult the doctor if they wished. During the year we made videos on breast self-examination and hysterectomy, spent £50 on books, and collected a variety of health education leaflets and addresses of various self-help and health interest groups. These were available for all women to see in the main room.

There were a number of difficulties in achieving our aims during the time I worked at the clinic, some of which resulted from how the clinic was started and others from the general practice setting. The awe in which most of us have been brought up to hold doctors is hard to banish completely. The volunteers, including myself, had some factual knowledge of women's health problems and experience and understanding of the emotional and social components of health but, when working in a clinic with one or two women doctors, there was always the temptation to refer to the 'medical expert'. Those with no specific health training felt less capable of providing women with information, yet those with training often felt unsure how to de-medicalise their work, impart knowledge, or help women who were depressed or anxious. Women themselves often used physical symptoms as their 'ticket' into the clinic, and it was easy for volunteers who were not confident in their counselling skills to collude with them and not explore more sensitive psychological areas. It was difficult to develop the self-help aspect of our work and to expand discussion of alternative therapies in a traditional general practice setting. Many of these problems might have been lessened had we spent more time together before the clinic opened. We could then have shared our ideas, skills and information, possibly anticipated some problems, and been clearer about how we would try to achieve our aims. As it was, we had no training sessions and, although we tried to meet monthly at first and later weekly, volunteers from outside the health centre found it difficult to attend all meetings and missed the informal contact from which those in the centre benefited. Because access to the clinic was restricted to patients registered with the practice, on average only four women attended each session. Although they were able to have time to talk, some of the volunteers felt under-used and it was not easy to generate enthusiasm for new developments. The small numbers also precluded setting up self-help groups.

There were, nevertheless, many very positive aspects to the work. Firstly, all women who attended the clinic were pleased to be able to talk to another woman. Many came because they had been unable to approach their male GP about their symptoms and some had been referred by their male GP, who recognised that his patient would find it easier to talk to a woman, and that she needed more time than he had to offer. Muslim women and those with breast or sexual problems particularly sought out the clinic. The informal atmosphere helped many women to feel more relaxed and able to talk openly or cry, and the availability of the creche gave some mothers the only space for themselves during the day. The clinic also provided reassurance for women with long-standing problems that they were not 'neurotic' or 'demanding'. By taking a more holistic view of their health, it was clear why conventional drug-orientated therapy was inappropriate and ineffective on its own, and we were able to legitimise their problems rather than dismiss them as 'psychosomatic'. This often helped women who wanted to stop taking drugs, especially tranquillisers, to do so. The books and leaflets were a popular and useful resource for local women, many of whom could not affort to buy them or did not know where to find them. There was a special interest in diet, relaxation, and general anatomy and physiology.

Women brought a wide range of issues and symptoms to the clinic. There were those we expected – contraception, sexual problems, the menopause, cystitis and thrush, depression and period problems – but the number of women specifically express-ing fears of breast cancer surprised us. There were women with severe medical problems which had not been picked up before, often because the woman had been too embarrassed to report her symptoms. Some women had severe emotional problems requir-ing more than counselling, but we also talked to women who were in difficult and often violent relationships, were incest survivors, or had spent years on tranquillisers or sleeping pills.

I feel that what most women were asking for was a little more time to discuss their worries and for more information about their bodies and about drugs or surgical procedures they might be advised to accept, so they could make choices and take more control over their health. As an illustration I shall describe some of the women who came to the clinic.

Women who came to the clinic

Jane came asking for a cervical smear but said she was interested in talking generally about her health. It soon became clear that she was afraid of an internal examination and of intercourse. She had had one internal examination – describing the speculum as 'that silver gun' – so her previous experience can be imagined! She had been married six months but had very little idea of her own anatomy or of how to express her sexuality. During three visits we looked at diagrams and a model of the female reproductive organs and genital area. She also examined a speculum and we both wished there was a better instrument for the job. She asked many questions, and together we worked out how she would like to control the pace of the doctor's examination and how she could relax. This discussion led on to her sexual needs. She was tense, her husband too fast and intercourse was painful. She did not know whether it would be possible to change the situation and, if so, in what way. We discussed again her need for control over what she felt was an invasion of her body, and we also talked about her need for closeness, wanting to give pleasure to her husband, and her right to receive pleasure and understanding from him. At the same time, I hope I gave her the chance to talk about any previous traumatic sexual experiences or doubts she might have had about whether she wanted to stay with her husband. We went together to see the female GP and Jane was able to ask the doctor to go slowly. Then she looked at her own cervix using a mirror and torch. She should feel more confident next time she sees a doctor and hopefully be able to talk to her husband about her sexual needs. She also knows that there are books that she can read and that there are women who are willing to support her in what she is trying to do.

Surinder's three young children accompanied her to the clinic and played in the creche. Surinder herself was very quiet and depressed, and said she had no-one to talk to except her health visitor and felt trapped. She is a Muslim and only wanted to talk to women. She suffered from migraines and insomnia, her husband was an alcoholic, and they had very little money. He was often violent towards her but she felt she could not leave, as neither her family nor his would support her or the children, and she would be isolated from her community. Although I could not offer Surinder solutions, I was able to help her express her unhappiness and anger. She talked to the doctor about her physical symptoms, and they both understood that her poor physical health resulted mainly from her social and economic conditions. She was introduced to a worker from the Asian Women's Refuge who gave her information about this, and she said she felt much less isolated in knowing there was support if she did leave home. It was important that Surinder was able to talk in her first language to another woman from a similar cultural background, for there were inevitably many issues she found hard to express in English and whose significance I would not realise. I was also unable to judge how realistic were her expectations of how her family would react to her situation.

Judith visited the clinic to ask for advice about the contraceptive pill after there had been publicity about its possible long-term effects. During our discussion of the changes she noticed in her body during her menstrual cycle, she mentioned changes in breast size. I asked if she examined her breasts but she said she was so frightened of what she might find that she never did this. I am sure most women have conflicting emotions over this, and I myself vacillate between regular examinations and then months without doing so. The fear of having to have a mastectomy if I find a lump paralyses me.

At the clinic there is no expert and client in these discussions. I may understand the pathology of breast cancer and have epidemiological information about its incidence or five-year survival rates, but this knowledge plays little part in the feelings I share with the woman about changes in body image, fear of cancer, death and loss of sexuality. Women I talk to often feel guilty because they have been told by the medical profession they must examine their own breasts. They need the space to talk about their fears and ambivalence, and come to their own decisions about what to do. This is the type of issue I would like raised in training sessions for Well Women Clinic workers, for I think it promotes a more equal relationship between women patients and health workers from which both benefit.

Melanie had begun her menopause and was suffering from hot flushes and back pain. She had read about Hormone Replacement Therapy (HRT) in a magazine and wanted to know more about it. I asked Melanie how much she understood about the menopause and gave her some more information. I also showed her some books about the menopause and talked over things she could do to alleviate her symptoms, including changes in her diet. Then we talked a little about the 'pros and cons' of HRT, and I suggested she see the woman doctor who had a special interest in menopausal problems and then make up her own mind. She agreed to this, and they both came to the conclusion that it was not suitable for her. I felt Melanie should have the opportunity of the best-informed medical opinion as well as support if she was unhappy with what the doctor recommended. I also tried to see how the changes in her body were affecting her emotionally, and she talked about the fear of growing old and of feeling 'redundant' now her children had left home. Melanie visited the clinic a number of times to tell me how she was managing her hot flushes and to talk about the future. She had enjoyed reading about other women's experiences of growing old and realising that there was 'life after 50'! She also talked about how difficult it was to try to change her diet, to find the new ingredients, not to be able to afford more expensive bread, and to persuade her husband to change his eating habits – all factors I sometimes forget. I was pleased she felt she could legitimately visit the clinic without the entrance ticket of physical symptoms.

The future

Many people at some time in their lives benefit from being able to share their anxieties with a sympathetic listener. Our emotions intimately affect our physical health but, for most people with emotional problems, there is no middle ground between seeing the doctor for a five-minute appointment where the discussion is likely to be limited to physical symptoms and being sent to a psychiatrist to be 'diagnosed' (and often again given drug therapy). The popularity of the Samaritans, Cruise, radio advice programmes or 'Agony Aunt' columns testifies to people's needs to have impartial listeners. I believe that Well Women's Clinics can provide that middle point for women. From my experiences and what I have read and heard from other clinics, I have concluded that the best place for such clinics is outside a 'health' establishment and based in the community. Given the power of the medical establishment, it is almost impossible to de-medicalise health within a medical setting. If women can see that ordinary women with an interest in health and with some training and sharing of skills can set up a resource centre and listen sympathetically to their worries, they are much more likely to believe in their own abilities to change and control their health.

Whether or not a woman doctor should be present is a question I still find problematic. Only 20 per cent of GPs are women and I think all women should have the right to consult a female doctor. However, doctors are not renowned for imparting knowledge to their patients, for their counselling skills or for challenging the veneration we bestow on them and working collectively to redress the balance of power between them, other health workers and patients. I would rather see Well Women's Clinics run on a collective basis in a community, involving local women, and having no limits on access. General practice should be improved by increasing the proportion of female doctors, and by all doctors being more understanding of women's specific health problems. I think our clinic provided a valuable service to its women patients but was too wasteful of resources because it was limited to a selected population. Perhaps one or two surgeries a week, advertised as specifically for women who wanted to talk to a woman doctor with twenty minute or longer appointment slots, might be a compromise. A Well Women's Centre able to attract larger numbers of women would allow self-help groups to be developed, campaigns to be built for improved NHS and other local facilities – for example for black women or single mothers – and women's health courses to be run.

What's been in it for me

I have benefited personally from the work I have done: helping others has helped me to understand my own emotions and define my own needs.The generalised anger I used to feel about the oppression of women has been redirected into positive and more effective channels. At the same time, I have been able to come to terms with my own experiences of sexual violence. The issues raised through this work have certainly challenged my relationship with my male lover – and our relationship is all the better for it.

I have learnt skills and acquired knowledge that I did not have before. I joined a women's self-help therapy group and later completed a counselling diploma course, and now I feel more self-confident and am also better able to control my own health. I have changed my diet, I am more questioning of medical 'expertise', and I am beginning to see links between my own emotional and physical health but still have far to go.

There has also been the fun and excitement of sharing experiences, of giving talks to which women have responded with warmth and appreciation, and of seeing women overcoming immense personal difficulties and then starting to believe in themselves and their own capacity to change and survive. I am still frustrated and angry – the pace of change is too slow for me. But the pleasures and strengths of sisterhood are powerful and help to sustain me.

Acknowledgements

To the women who phoned Rape Crisis and visited the Well Women's Clinic and shared their fears and sadness, hopes and laughter; to all the women at Rape Crisis, especially Ros, Hilary and Helen; to my fellow workers at the clinic and practice especially Joan, Clare and Paul; to Judith, Mary, Maggie, Jane, Mel and Pauline for challenges and inspiration – you have all 'open-eyed' me. Thank you.

Thank you, Shirley and Christine, for helping me with my appalling grammar and spelling.

Love and gratitude to all my friends for your care and support, and to Dave for always being there, even when the going was rough.

Useful Addresses

Women's Health Information Centre: 52 Featherstone Street, London EC 1.
    01–251 6580
London Rape Crisis Centre: PO Box 69, London WC1X 9NJ. 01–837 1600
    (will give numbers of nearest Rape Crisis Centre)

References

Brownmiller S (1977) *Against Our Will – Men, Women and Rape*. Harmonds-
    worth: Penguin
Doyal L *et al* (1983) *Cancer in Britain – The Politics of Prevention*. London:
    Pluto Press
Phillips A & Rakusen J (1980) *Our Bodies, Ourselves*. Harmondsworth:
    Penguin
Rogers C R (1967) *On Becoming a Person*. London: Constable
The London Rape Crisis Centre (1984) *Sexual Violence – The Reality for
    Women*. London: The Women's Press

9

Child Abuse: Are Abusing Women Abused Women?

BIE NIO ONG

About the Author

See Chapter 2.

Ideas about child rearing are forever changing, and these changing ideas influence the practice of mothers and those who advise them. We have, for example, the ideas of Bowlby, who argued that the infant should experience a warm, intimate and continuous relationship with the mother, and his theory of 'maternal deprivation' was very influential in the 1950s and 60s (Bowlby 1953). The impact of child psychology in those years was enormous and many professionals such as health visitors tailored their advice to mothers according to these theories. Early expert advice in the area of child rearing generally advocated a 'scientific' approach (Ehrenreich & English 1979).

The development of expert advice has continued to the present day, based on the twin assumptions that, on the one hand, women instinctively know what to do with their children and, on the other hand, need the guidance of experts. Of course, there is a profound contradiction between those two assumptions and women suffer as a result.

In the 1980s, the leading 'expert' book is Penelope Leach's *Baby and Child from Birth to Five* (Leach 1977) which shows all the hallmarks of the trend to centre on the needs of the child and to be an 'earth mother'. Leach homes in on the feelings of the child, the mother's feelings as a carer, and the book claims to avoid prescription and not to lay down any rules. Yet there is a powerful underlying rule that motherhood (she hardly discusses parenthood) means making a child happy. The image of the ideal mother is one who sacrifices, who puts the child's needs – both physical and emotional – first. This approach is very seductive, as the image of motherhood is a woman who is raising a well-developed, emotionally balanced child who is living proof of her success as a mother.

My main argument is that how motherhood is portrayed in the literature – and this of course reflects the dominant ideas in our society – abuses women as people. The demands on women as mothers have to be analysed in terms of their personal development as individuals, and not just in terms of how children develop. My view of child abuse is different from the widely accepted idea that women who have been abused themselves as children in turn reproduce that abuse when they have their own children. I do not intend to reiterate that argument, but rather to focus on what being a mother means for women. I argue that 'the institution of motherhood' (Rich 1977) is stifling for women, it suffocates them, and makes it very difficult to be the self-effacing, caring and giving people they are expected to be. Because motherhood does not allow women to grow as persons in their own right, the potential of 'ideal' motherhood is hard to fulfil. Moreover, material and cultural circumstances can facilitate or prohibit the growth of this potential, and the case studies I shall give later in the chapter will illustrate this.

The other side of the Leach picture of motherhood is described by Tillie Olsen:

> 'But from those years she had to manage, old humiliations and terrors rose up ... The children's needings; the grocer's face or this merchant's wife she had had to beg credit from when credit was a disgrace ...; school coming, and the desperate going over the old to see what could yet be remade; the soups of meat bones begged "for the dog" one winter...'
> (Olsen 1980, p 78).

This chapter, therefore, discusses the myths and realities of motherhood, and the views and expectations women have of themselves. Within this context I shall discuss the occurrence – *not* the causality – of child abuse. Women who feel deeply abused in their personal growth cannot allow their children the space to grow, and some women resort to abuse. In this sense I want to turn the commonly-posed question of 'why do certain women abuse their children?' on its head, and pose the alternative question of 'why do more women not abuse their children?'

Some aspects of motherhood

Women in contemporary western society are seen as the lynchpin of the family. As wives they care for their husbands, as mothers they care for their children, as daughters they care for their parents, and as members of an 'extended' family they care for relatives (Finch & Groves 1983). In practice, most women care at least for a husband and children because just over half of British families are 'nuclear' families (Rapoport *et al.* 1982) – and certain notions of women's work have emerged as a result. Women's work involves domestic work and child care, and emotional support of husband and children is seen as part and parcel of that work. Women themselves, in carrying out the tasks of caring, are expected to 'cope'. In particular, women as mothers are expected to be copers. They are individuals who can handle the pressures of life calmly and effectively: 'The more successful a mother is, the less apparent her presence becomes as she moves unobtrusively through the home, contending quietly with the demands of housework, husband and children. In other words, to cope successfully is to deny yourself a voice: the best mother is one who is seen but not heard.' (Graham 1982, p 105).

Many feminists have discussed the oppression of women within the home and their submission and passivity in relation to the division of labour between the sexes (Oakley 1974; Rowbotham 1976). But there is another side to this – women's power as mothers. Children are predominantly brought up in small units, be they nuclear families or single parent families, and are also considered as their parents' property. This has profound repercussions for the relationship between mother and child.

> 'A mother's influence is greatest when there is no alternative
> and no escape. For the first time in history this has become the
> situation for the majority of mothers and children in society
> ... The result is that today's mother probably has total power
> over her child, and over no one and nothing else. He is
> exposed to the full impact of her personality.' (Dally 1982, p
> 201)

There is thus an apparent contradiction between women as powerless and low in status, and women as holders of power over their children. It is precisely this contradiction which is the key to explaining women's violence towards their children. Women are relatively excluded from the public sphere of life which is dominated by men and male values of work, politics and power; women's domain is the private, which consists of the family and caring. Recently, discussions have taken place about the relationship between the public and the private, and how female servicing supports male power (Garmarnikov *et al.* 1983) but I shall focus on women's power in the private sphere of motherhood. As the principal carers of children, women determine their children's destiny to a great extent and thereby exercise power. Children, on the other hand, call this power continually into question, thus undermining women as mothers (Ong 1985).

In present day Britain the promotion of family values and family life is particularly strong. In spite of public statements to the contrary, Mrs Thatcher and her government create a political, economic and cultural climate which pushes women more and more in to the home and idealises women's role as mother. At the same time these policies create materially adverse conditions for families and for women within them. The system of state benefits is one example where women are forced to cope with caring with a minimum level of support, and women in time of recession shoulder an enormous burden of work. The combination of the material and ideological aspects of motherhood in our society create the oppressive context in which many women are mothering their children.

I argue that the economic, social and psychological pressures upon women which precipitate child abuse make it impossible to see child abuse as an individual problem. In order to understand individual experiences, we have to analyse the wider context and confront the issue of the violence of the institution of motherhood. Women as mothers are violated in their personal growth because they are expected to cope, no matter what the circumstances. In talking with women about their experiences as mothers, I hope to illustrate the relationship between violence *to* mothers and *by* mothers.

My analysis is rather different from that of the National Society for the Prevention of Cruelty to Children (NSPCC). Their model of mothers abusing their children has been very influential in professional circles, and stresses a psychological analysis of the problem: '... our mothers were simply not equipped as people to cope effectively with the task of child rearing. A basic lack of motherliness as a feature of abusive parents has been well documented in the literature and our impressions tend to confirm this as being central to the problem of abuse.' (NSPCC 1976, pp 87–89).

An important strand in this analysis is the definition of the problem as an individual one. Of course there are individual problems, but the social context in which abuse takes place is equally important. The focus on the individual results from practitioners' concern to remedy an anomalous situation. However, the realisation that motherhood is a socially constructed concept is important in order to understand the societal pressures which bear upon individual women to succeed as mothers.

On a very practical level, this means that professionals dealing with women who abuse their children have to look closely at their own attitudes and beliefs about motherhood. They need to ask themselves whether they subscribe to the dominant notions of mothers as carers, as people who cope and who are child-centred, or whether they understand the oppression of mothers as people who sacrifice, who struggle against adverse conditions, who suffer. It is crucially important for professional practice to understand what models of motherhood underlie that practice.

In presenting some case studies, I hope to illustrate that alternative conceptions of motherhood can be therapeutic in the sense that they direct practice away from individualised problem-solving to group-oriented solidarity.

The research

In a study at an NSPCC Centre, in-depth interviews took place with women who had abused their children or were suspected of having abused or 'allowed' abuse. In those interviews the issues discussed included family background, pregnancy and childbirth, attitudes and feelings towards the target child, general ideas about parenting, financial and housing situation and relationships with the NSPCC. Following discussions in the research team on feminist research methodologies (Roberts 1980), we carried out the interviews on a more reciprocal basis than conventional social research recommends.

In traditional interview methods the relationship between interviewer and interviewee is unequal, with the interviewer in charge, asking questions and directing a conversation, and the interviewee as the passive information-provider. Feminists have criticised this approach as being unsuitable to research that wants to find out what people really feel and experience. They argue that the best 'results' are achieved if the relationship is non-hierarchical and when the interviewer is prepared to invest her personal identity in the relationship (Oakley 1981).

In our research we worked in this way but, as we were dealing with powerful emotions such as those surrounding child abuse, our involvement had to be strongly supportive and empathetic towards the interviewees. Sometimes, the boundaries between in-depth interviewing and therapy were difficult to draw. All the interviews inevitably had some element of painful disclosure, and this had to be handled by the women and the interviewer. We accepted that in certain cases an overlap of interviewing and therapy would occur because with the kind of research method we used – which involved a relationship built up over four months – this was possible. The interviewer took 'responsibility' for what she had stirred up, and in all interviews she was able to resolve this with the woman in question. Social workers and the staff of the Family Centre were, of course, available if necessary.

The interview data is largely qualitative in character, as my interest was primary women's own experiences. The wealth of data also helps in understanding the relationship between dominant ideas of motherhood in our society, and how women respond to these in their day-to-day lives. An explanation of women's feelings and thought processes provides an important link between those ideas and reality. Therefore I relied on women's accounts of the pressures of motherhood, and I shall let the women speak for themselves.

Did we choose motherhood?

In our society it is assumed that all women want to be mothers at some stage in their lives. Many women do not ask the question 'why children?' (Dowrick & Grundberg 1980) and the women I interviewed were no exception to this. The majority had had children while they were still teenagers. In contemporary Britain, and in many western countries, the recession is biting deep and unemployment is rising, especially for young people. Many of the young women I talked to were implicitly or explicitly aware of the limited chances they had of an independent, economically viable future. The promotion of the family as the caring unit was seductive, especially the idea of romantic love and babies, and so they had babies at an early age in the hope of achieving these ideals. However reality often caught up with them in a short space of time, when they had to confront financial hardship, unsupportive relationships with partners and their lost youth.

Debbie, for example, wanted to be sterilised now that she had three children, of whom one was in care. She said,

> Debbie: 'Yes, I'll be better off because I don't want any more. Even if it didn't work out between my husband and me, I

still wouldn't have any if I got married again. I wasn't
meant for kids, really.'
BNO: 'What makes you say that?'
Debbie: 'No, I wasn't. It's just not me.'
BNO: 'Do you feel that that is you, or do you want to do other
things?'
Debbie: 'I think, it's because I haven't done much. I mean, I
was only seventeen when I had Lorna.'

Debbie and other women in the study could not recall having
chosen to become mothers, and they talked about getting 'caught'.
In spite of not having planned their pregnancies all these women
accepted becoming a mother as their natural destiny. In that sense
they felt it was counterproductive to dwell on feelings of regret,
yet they often said things like 'I'm rushing my life past' or 'I could
have had a life for myself'.

The women attempted to reconstruct the past in positive terms; for
example they considered having a baby as achieving a valued
status. As avenues for building up some sort of career are largely
blocked, becoming a mother is considered an appropriate way to
become respected as an adult and as someone who contributes to
society. Some of the women entered a 'competition' to have babies
as young as possible. Gillian said proudly:

'There was my friend Doreen, she had a baby first. Then it
was me, and the rest after me.'

This pride at being the first often turned into something to be
regretted, because friends turned away when they did not understand the routines of looking after a small baby. Pressures of lack
of money and cramped accommodation made the romantic ideal
fall apart. Material circumstances forced the women to change
their ideas about love and motherhood, and when discussing their
present predicament they did not paint a picture in fairy tale
terms. Some women were very bitter about their partners, who
did not behave as the 'prince on a white horse', and complained
about their material circumstances, but others could only be
fatalistic:

Woman: 'I don't know really. I'll just keep carrying on like I do
everyday.'
BNO: 'Just live from day to day?'
Woman: 'Yes.'
BNO: 'And hope things get better?'
Woman: 'Somehow, I don't think they will get better.'

These different responses of bitterness or a fatalistic outlook on
life can be understood when we look at the discrepancy between

ideas about marriage and family life as portrayed in novels, the media and government publications, and the grim reality of many British families (Townsend 1979; Graham 1984).

Being a mother and housewife

Ann Oakley was the first sociologist to study systematically the combination of the two roles of a woman as a domestic worker and a child-rearer. These two jobs make the working week of a woman very long, and in a sense they contradict each other. Housework is short-term and repetitive, child-care has a single long-term goal, and a 'successful' mother brings up her children to do without her (Oakley 1974, p 167).

The women in our study all combined the two roles and their burden was seldom alleviated because they did not have partners who were prepared to share some of the work. In the families we studied, the sexual division of labour was strict. The women were the carers and the men the providers and, even though men were often unemployed, this division was maintained. Most women were living on a shoestring, and this meant that their tasks of housekeeping and child-care were even more arduous. They had to put in extra labour to make ends meet, for example, by mending clothes, or going round shops looking for bargains.

The support women received from relatives or neighbours was often limited and they were rarely freed from the bonds of child-care. There was thus little space to satisfy their own adult needs. At the same time the women's own attitudes about substitute child-care were negative. If it was not possible for a member of the family or a friend to look after their children, they chose to do it themselves rather than have professional care. The issue was not money, because the nurseries they could have used were subsidised. It was the discrepancy in values which was more important. This became clear when discussing the work methods of the NSPCC nursery staff compared with the women's own ways of handling their children. Kate said:

> 'I mean, if he does something naughty like, at the dinner table, when he walks away from the dinner table. They (nursery staff) just tell him off. I'd smack him for it, because he doesn't do it at home, and he gets away with murder here, which I don't like at all.'

Recalling the underlying values of Penelope Leach, it is clear that the nursery staff subscribe to these, while the mothers are more concerned with discipline than individual self-expression. Lillian Breslow Rubin (1976) discusses the concern with discipline in the working class and relates that directly to their material conditions. Because they experience life at the bottom of the class system, they see discipline as a better strategy for a way out, and do not feel that they can afford to let their children explore their individuality. It is considered more important to behave well and make progress at school by studying hard than to develop self-expression and creativity. Achievement may lead on to a better job and more secure material future but self-development is not likely to pay off in this way. All this is understandable against the background of constrained financial and material conditions.

Thus the theory and practice of professionals who are promoting child-centred expressiveness cannot be followed by women who find those values threatening to their own values and existence. It is important that professionals examine whether their ideas are accepted by their clients because, if there is a wide divergence or even conflict between the two points of view, no collaboration is possible.

The other side of disciplining relates to the question of women's power over children. Discipline is a visible sign of control over children, and is seen as a measure of success as a child-rearer. However, in a situation of isolation this control can get out of hand and turn into child abuse.

Women's isolation within the home (Rowbotham 1976), the expectations that women will cope, and the dismissal of their complaints by partners and professionals (GPs who say that it is normal for a young mother to pop Valium) all contribute to a growing frustration in women. Most of the women we talked to referred to their isolation and saw it as a major factor in their violence towards their children. Often it was discipline getting out of control, or losing your temper and 'forgetting yourself'.

> 'He (husband) was drinking – no support at all. And in the night it was me up, up, and the kids were up at five in the morning. So, I reached out for help. I was asking the welfare for help for a long time. I didn't get any help. Nobody came . . . So, I coped for another three months. Then I hit Eddy. I just snapped . . . I just smacked him across the face and then somebody reported me, that I was beating him up.'

She felt that she had coped so long, without any recognition of the pressures she was under. As she had no avenues of release for her growing frustration because she was isolated in the home, she took it out on her child. In a way he embodied the main factor which kept her bound to the house, and he was an available target.

Women's confinement to the house can result in different strategies for dealing with their children. The one Wendy 'chose' illustrates the uncontrollable anger and frustration; another is a laissez-faire approach. This implies not entering into any conflict with children, but just letting them do what they want and leaving the disciplining to someone else, often the male partner. However, this strategy can also bring violence into existence. In probably half of the reported cases of child abuse, the main perpetrators are men. This could be partly explained by the fact that in many households men are allocated the role of disciplinarian. In those cases where the woman has retreated from disciplining children as the burden of housework, care and other tasks require all her energy, men may react by exaggerating their role. For example, Gillian tells the following story:

> *Gillian*: 'He does all the disciplining, I don't do it at all, even now.'
> *BNO*: Do you hit the children?'
> *Gillian*: 'I do, but I don't hurt her like he does. I mean, when he hits them, he really hits them. With me, I just tap them and she still plays up all the time.'
> *BNO*: 'What do you feel works then?'
> *Gillian*: 'It worries me and makes me depressed and upset, because he hurts her. He gets all the discipline, you know, anything he wants her to do, she'll do it, do it for him. But with me, she won't do it, she just plays up all the time.'

Gillian's husband finds her a 'softie' and thinks harsh punishment is the answer. Gillian has no other answer to him than being upset. She feels subordinate to his wishes, and has little power to change the division of labour. Within this climate, control over children can be easily distorted and difficult to alter.

Women's own identities

Many women who have become mothers cease to have a clear self-identity separate from their role as mothers. In many cultures a woman's status as child bearer has been the test of her woman-hood (Rich 1977). This means that for many women being a woman becomes equated with being a mother. Moreover, publicly women are expected to value motherhood positively, and if they feel negative about being a mother they either keep it to them-selves, or air their feelings only in trusted private circles (Ong,

1983). Against this background, it is no wonder that many of the women interviewed found the question 'how do you see yourself?' surprising. They reacted often with bewilderment, and said things like 'I don't understand'. Being a mother appeared to be the over-riding factor, and answers such as the following were typical:

> 'Totally a mother ... I think there's three categories: the kids come first, their enjoyment, their breakfast, tea, everything. Dave comes second, and if I want anything, I come last. It's always the kids first.'

Apart from two women who had reservations about identifying with the mother role, all women presented the picture of motherhood as a sacrifice. This reflects clearly the dominant values in our society that women are first and foremost mothers (Dowrick & Grundberg 1980). However, the way in which the question was asked could have contributed to the stereotyped way the answers were given. Throughout the interviews it became clear that there were cracks beneath the surface, and the main manifestation of this was self-destruction. The pressure to cope with the role of mother is very strong, both from society and the immediate environment and from within the woman herself. Admitting that you have sacrificed your own identity is too difficult, and blaming yourself for failing and getting depressed seems to be one way out. Gillian said this:

> '... and I was still getting depressed, and the doctor came back to see me and he said 'you're not well at all. I think you'd better come into hospital' because I wasn't sleeping properly. I only had a few hours at night and then got up and was working. The things I didn't need to do every day I just left it. I didn't put cups away and pots away. I just left them because I couldn't do it. I was too weak and tired. He (doctor) said "what you need, young lady, is to go to hospital and have a short rest". So I went in and they sorted me out.'

Gillian's strategy is to legitimise her 'not coping' by translating it into a medical framework. She finds it more difficult to question the sexual division of labour between her and her husband, or to alter the demanding behaviour of her children, because she would have to be clear about her own individual needs. Instead, she reverts to 'illness'. Her strategy is acceptable, for in our society the tendency to medicalise non-medical problems is widespread (Illich 1979). Especially for women this medicalisation is a logical extension of their 'natural' being: emotionally unstable, weak, governed by biology (menstruation, reproductive cycle) (Jordanova 1980). To be 'ill' is acceptable but to be a 'non-coper' is not. By adopting the sick role, she can also be absolved from responsibility and can lean on others:

> '... being on my own with the two kids, that's what got me depressed. I had no one to help me or cope with the kids ... My friend went to see the psychiatrist you know, to sort my problems out and why I was getting depressed and how she could help me. And he said, "she needs a lot of friends, she needs people to come down and see her and she wants to get out more often." And she put her foot down (confronted the husband) and took me out.'

Thus, becoming ill serves several purposes: Gillian can be absolved from responsibility because she is ill, others take her complaints seriously and assume responsibility for her life, and she can challenge the sexual division of labour indirectly by proving that her burden of work makes her ill. However, by adopting this strategy she remains powerless, and fundamental changes are unlikely to take place.

There are major problems related to this 'illness' behaviour as opposed to 'not coping' behaviour. The idea that mothers 'are being seen but not heard' (Graham 1982) is widely accepted, and the women we interviewed referred often to a self-image of 'the one who comes last'. This concept leads to a disbelief in 'not coping', perpetuated by both the women themselves and the professionals who deal with them. In cases of breakdown, such as child abuse, professionals attempt to restore women to a position in which they can cope again with the demands of motherhood. By doing this, the origins of 'failure' in both material and ideological circumstances are not properly understood. Mothers are copers, and those who are not are failing as individuals. Allowing the labels 'bad', 'inadequate' or 'sick' to be put on women individualises the problem and leaves the women with feelings of guilt and shattered self-confidence (Chesler 1974). Instead, professionals should examine how motherhood is defined and how the notion of coping itself is oppressive and pathological. In view of the structural and material circumstances in which many women have to carry out their mothering role, it is no wonder that they break under the strain: how can we expect someone to cope, living in a one-bedroomed house with two children, with no support from her partner and little money to spend?

I am not arguing for a simplistic economistic model which overlooks people's personal responsibility. One cannot avoid focusing on the individuals concerned, but I want to move away from labelling them as 'deviant'. Of course, the question why some people abuse their children and others do not remains difficult to answer. Yet it is important to realise that the institution of motherhood, and the demands connected with it, calls violence into existence because women are violated in their personal development. An approach which takes into account both cultural values and individual problems is more useful in understanding child abuse.

Violence to children

All the women we interviewed were suspected of having abused their children, or having 'allowed' others (male partners) to abuse them. There was one case of a child who was suspected to be at risk, but had not actually been abused. We discussed with the women how they came to the attention of the NSPCC.

The most interesting feature in their own accounts is that all the women saw child abuse as an isolated event in their lives, totally unconnected with the usual pattern of interaction with their children or in their family as a whole. They also did not relate their own perceptions of the pressures of motherhood to the occurrence of violence to their children. Thus, most of the women described the reason why they were noticed by the NSPCC as a one-off accident:

> 'We were arguing and fighting and the baby was clobbered off him, so I took him to the hospital and he ended up with a fractured skull, and he was screaming and that's when the NSPCC got in contact with us.'

As a result, women saw the Family Centre not as a place where they had to look at their own life and attitudes, or that of their partners. Their idea in coming to the centre was to get relief from their daily duties and from their children, who are looked after by professional nursery staff. On the one hand, this attitude is understandable considering the circumstances in which most of them live. On the other hand, the Family Centre aims to show women alternative forms of parenting and so create a space in which they can experiment with relationships with their children. However, most of the women were very resistant to these objectives. They were quite clear that what they needed from staff was support, advice and emotional back-up. Chris voices her needs unambiguously:

'Before I started coming here, you know, all my problems and that, with bills and things like that, I didn't know you could go to the gas place and say "I'll pay off so much a week" and I didn't know you could get so much help as I can now. Like when I'm in here and I have got a problem or something, or something is worrying me, I just tell the social worker and she helps me out.'

It is important to help people to improve their material conditions, as these can be a major factor in their oppressive predicament. Yet, at the same time social workers and other professionals are well aware of the problems of dependence and relinquishing responsibility. Most of the women were very adept at using those strategies, thereby avoiding the more fundamental issues of their violence, or their partners' violence towards their children.

In the interviews it was difficult to address directly the question of child abuse. As has become clear from the quotations, the women presented themselves according to what they felt was 'normal', namely being a concerned, sacrificing, coping mother. Child abuse was a 'freak' incident, not fitting into the normal pattern of daily life. It was either something to be explained as unaccountable behaviour because they were depressed, or as a one-off incident beyond their responsibility. I would argue that their accounts are not deliberately misleading or untrue. The women's interpretations of their own lives make those explanations quite logical. They see their existence as an isolated, individual one – not embedded in society as a whole – and therefore their abuse is their personal problem. They cannot see any broader, less individualised explanation. Because of this highly individualised 'failure', their resistance to change is high as well. They also realise that any change would have to take place against a background of adverse conditions. Understanding these perceptions can be the first step in the direction of alternative ways of professional intervention.

De-individualising the problem

The women's movement has developed the concept of 'sisterhood', meaning solidarity and collective action (Dalley 1983). This concept could be useful in building an alternative practice which aims at de-individualising child abuse. If women were stimulated to share their experiences of mothering, to analyse the pressures they are under and recognise their common features, they would be making a start in breaking out of a cycle of individual guilt and failure. However, for many women this would mean starting a revolution. Especially in situations where they feel under surveillance, like being at the NSPCC, self-preservation seems to be instinctive. Many of the women at the Family Centre resisted the idea of talking to each other about personal and problematic issues. Examples like this were given:

> 'I mean, I don't (talk with others). It's like when your child does something and a mother is sat there and she'll say "Oh, my baby did that as well". But you don't have to compete, I don't think you have to compete.'

and

> 'I've been through it myself, I don't know. I've got my life, my own kids, that's all I'm worried about. People think I'm heartless, but I've been through it all, and I'm hard now. I couldn't care less. I've got my kids.'

In a situation where everyone feels they have to 'prove' that they are good mothers, it is difficult to change feelings of distrust. Many of the women conveyed an impression that they would not trust others to keep information confidential, not to be competitive, or not to 'get back at me'. This level of distrust was to some extent a self-fulfilling prophecy of not giving trust and therefore not receiving any.

At the same time, there was a realisation that one could be supported by others in the same predicament. Some were very careful and limited this to purely practical help, as this woman did:

> 'I had a problem, the little boy was getting on my nerves and he wouldn't go to sleep and then they said "why don't you put some gel on his teeth?" and we help each other that way.'

Very few women felt safe enough to cross that boundary and 'open up' in more personal ways. It was notable that conversations appeared to the researchers to discuss profound issues such as relationships, having been abused themselves, or other such topics, yet the women themselves appeared to interpret those conversations differently. They seemed to feel that they were relating stories to each other but not revealing their true feelings. Thus, on the whole, sharing of experiences did not take place. Mandy is an exception when she says:

> *Mandy*: 'Well, sometimes I tell the mothers about my problems, but again, they are just like mine.'
> *BNO*: 'In what sense?'

> *Mandy*: 'Well, they feel, well, sometimes they feel it's hard to cope with their kids.'
> *BNO*: 'Does that give you a bit of strength, to know that some people have the same problems?'
> *Mandy*: 'Yes, because I know I'm not on my own.'

This realisation of 'not being on your own' is an important starting point for working with these women, and some of the social workers have been developing group work within the NSPCC setting.

Of course, there are important contradictions for social workers and other professionals who are dealing with both the parents and the children. The protection of children is a principal priority, especially in cases where the child has been proven to be seriously at risk. Then, the law poses its limitations in defining the problem. Where the abuser is the male partner, magistrates only accept the need to protect a child when they use phrases such as 'Mother failed to protect'. In terms of solidarity between mothers, this definition poses fundamental problems because it describes the issue in individual terms. Attempts to de-individualise child abuse have to confront these limitations in legal terms and working practices. Moreover, the dilemma between the interests of the parents – for example, their personal development – and the interests of the child – its physical and emotional safety – cannot be easily resolved in present day social work practice. Yet, in spite of these very real difficulties, I feel that avenues do exist for exploring how to stimulate solidarity, shared insights and breakdown of isolated guilt.

While we were doing our research we had more room to experiment and take risks than social workers and other professionals who have a direct responsibility for their clients. We were therefore able to try alternative strategies. The first was to show each woman the video-recordings of a play session that she had had with her child. From the usual research perspective, this play session would be used to assess the quality of the relationship between mother and child. From the perspective of feminist research, it was also a tool to enable women to reflect on their own development. We therefore showed every woman her own video, with her social worker and head of the Family Centre present. The two professionals adopted a positive approach in the sense of discussing first of all the images of the videotape which opened up new potential for both the woman and her child to progress in their relationship. They created a non-threatening atmosphere in which the woman did not feel under surveillance, but was intrigued at seeing herself and was able to use the opportunity to reflect on her own and her child's behaviour. Instead of having to rely on retrospective accounts of an interaction between mother and child, or on observations which could not be repeated, the videos provided concrete evidence. In this way the videotapes were used to support on-going work by the social worker and the Family Centre. They could throw new light on old problems or reinforce certain issues that had already been under discussion. For the researcher they served the important function of giving the women something back, and providing the opportunity to see 'behind' the research (Oakley 1981).

The women brought their reflections on their individual video-recordings back to the group. Often they were couched in competitive terms – such as who looked best – or stayed at the level of excitement about having a film made about oneself. But there was a certain amount of sharing and attempts to work out what the tapes were saying to them.

The second strategy was to write a short paper for the women about the interviews, emphasising the similarity of experiences and the strength of sharing and support. The women then had a group discussion in which they tried to focus on these two topics, but they found it difficult to move away from their personal predicament, as if they were 'losing' something. They also attempted to identify each other in the descriptions and quotes.

Thus, there was a lot of competition between them, and showing off about who was most 'together' about mothering. Some women also showed a lot of suspicion towards each other. They read criticism of themselves into the text and tried to discover who had said these things. It became clear that there were 'vast spaces' between the researcher, social worker and head of the Family Centre on the one hand, and the women on the other, over the issue of sharing and sisterhood. The women did not give up their resistance to wanting to be individually-oriented rather than group-oriented. They said things like, 'No-one understands how I feel', and they found the idea of sisterhood alien, although they realised at the same time that there was some benefit in sharing.

The social workers had previously run some role-play sessions with the women, exploring their relationships in general and in particular those with their parents. These sessions had had some impact but this was limited, due to the women's resistance to going into issues in-depth and to sharing with each other. From these two experiences it becomes clear that a many-sided approach is needed. The paper, for example, could be a starting point for discussions, followed by role-play and video-taping, while individual therapy should continue to strengthen women's belief in themselves. Group and family therapy should run in parallel. This involves a multi-disciplinary approach, which is also very labour-intensive. It may not seem feasible in many settings, but the NSPCC does seem to have made in-roads into this sort of broader approach in some of their establishments.

Conclusion

In this chapter I have argued that in our society problems tend to be individualised, and child abuse is no exception to this. In order to move away from this tendency we have to understand how motherhood is defined, how it shapes women's existence, and how it violates women in their development as people. For professionals this means that they have to analyse their own ideas about motherhood, and confront the issue of their definitions of 'good' mothers. This involves a closer look at their practice, their priorities and interventions. Restoring women to being 'good' mothers does not take those issues into account and does not alter the social context in which many women mother. The 'natural order' has to be called into question in order to set goals which do not oppress women in their motherhood. One way forward could be to employ and develop in practice the concept of 'sisterhood', so that women can share experiences and support each other in understanding the pressures of mothering.

Acknowledgements

I should like to thank all the women who allowed me to interview them. The research was carried out as part of a SSRC funded project 'Abusing mothers and their children', Department of Psychology, Manchester University, 1982–1983.

References

Bowlby J (1953) *Child Care and the Growth of Love.* Harmondsworth: Penguin
Breslow Rubin L (1976) *Worlds of Pain.* New York: Basic Books
Chesler P (1974) *Women and Madness.* London: Allen Lane
Dalley G (1983) Ideologies of care: a feminist contribution to the debate. *Critical Social Policy,* **3** (2), 72–81

Dally A (1982) *Inventing Motherhood: The Consequences of an Ideal*. London: Burnett

Dowrich S & Grundberg S ed (1980) *Why Children?* London: Women's Press

Ehrenreich B & English D (1979) *For Her own Good*. London: Pluto Press

Finch J & Groves D (1983) *A Labour of Love*. London: Routledge & Kegan Paul

Garmarnikov E, Morgan D, Purvis J & Taylorson D eds (1983) *The Public and the Private*. London: Heinemann

Graham H (1982) Coping: or how mothers are seen and not heard. In Friedman S & Sarah E ed *On the Problem of Men*. London: Women's Press

Graham H (1984) *Women, Health and the Family*. Brighton: Wheatsheaf Books

Illich I (1979) *Limits to Medicine*. Harmondsworth: Penguin

Jordanova L (1980) Natural facts: a historical perspective on science and sexuality. In MacCormack C & Strathern M ed *Nature, Culture and Gender*. Cambridge: Cambridge University Press.

Leach P (1977) *Baby and Child from Birth to Five*. Harmondsworth: Penguin

NSPCC Battered Child Research Team (1976) *At Risk*. London: Routledge & Kegan Paul

Oakley A (1974) *The Sociology of Housework*. New York: Pantheon Books

Oakley A (1981) Interviewing women: a contradiction in terms. In *Doing Feminist Research*. London: Routledge & Kegan Paul.

Olsen T (1980) *Tell Me a Riddle*. London: Virago

Ong BN (1983) *Our Motherhood. Women's Accounts of Pregnancy, Childbirth and Health Encounters*. Family Service Units discussion paper, London

Ong BN (1985) The paradox of wonderful children: the case of child abuse. *Early Child Development and Care*, **20** (3), 3

Rapoport R, Fogarty M & Rapoport R (1982) *Families in Britain*. London: Routledge & Kegan Paul

Rich A (1977) *Of Woman Born*. London: Virago

Roberts H ed (1981) *Doing Feminist Research*. London: Routledge & Kegan Paul

Rowbotham S (1976) *Woman's Consciousness, Man's World*. Harmondsworth: Penguin

Townsend P (1979) *Poverty in the United Kingdom: A Survey of Household Resources and Standards of Living*. Harmondsworth: Penguin

10
Postscript
CHRISTINE WEBB

This book has been written by a group of feminists working as 'professionals' or volunteers in women's health care both inside and outside the National Health Service. We have tried to describe how we bring into our work the feminist ideas to which we are committed, but we also acknowledge the limitations in what we do and the dilemmas and contradictions we face.

We think it is essential to share resources with those we work with, and information is one of the most important of our contributions. If people have knowledge about their health, the range of treatments available to them, what are the advantages and possible side-effects of these treatments, and what progress they might expect to make, then they can choose to exercise control over their health if they wish to. Without this kind of information, they are forced to remain *patients* in the literal sense – passive receivers of what others think is good for them. In the context in which we write and work, these 'others' are mainly men – or women who have been trained to think according to masculine definitions of women's health and how people should be treated. This masculine 'scientific' perspective views a person principally as a disordered body whose malfunctions are isolated from the rest of social life, with its prescriptions of appropriate roles and behaviour for women and men.

Sharing knowledge is therefore sharing power, but it also requires a radically different relationship between health workers and clients. True sharing and demystification of technical jargon are only possible in an equal relationship in which neither partner has more rights or privileges than the other. This kind of sharing and equality allow open discussion and mutual questioning and challenging of opinions. Through these processes people develop confidence in their ability to understand and take charge of their own health.

Feminist health care seeks to show people that their problems are not unique to them, but are shared by many others in similar situations, and particularly amongst women. Sometimes this is achieved by giving information, but putting women in touch with others and helping to form groups for mutual support and self-help are other approaches drawn from the women's movement.

Changes are not all one-sided, however, for feminists working in these ways also gain knowledge and awareness of the kinds of problems their clients face and their needs for help and support. This consciousness-raising has effects both on workers' 'professional' and personal lives.

People trying to use feminist methods in their work need support too. Putting these ideas into practice inevitably challenges others in the work situation, and their reactions may vary from patronising amusement to overt hostility. Just as feminist health workers try to provide support for clients struggling to make decisions and change their lives and health, so they need to gain support for themselves and give it to their feminist colleagues.

If this makes putting feminist ideas into practice sound warm and cosy, it is not meant to. Nor do we intend to hark back to a romantic past when skilled women health practitioners worked in an atmosphere of sisterhood. Women have always played an important role in caring for others, but the reality was one in which poverty and ignorance caused a great deal of suffering and many treatments were not particularly effective. This situation has changed less than we may think.

Although we have talked throughout the book as if 'feminism' is a single approach and set of ideas shared by all who describe themselves as feminists, this is clearly a simplification. There are many different kinds of feminist ideas and people incorporate them into their work in different ways. At the same time, the different contexts in which we work mean that opportunities to use alternative working styles vary enormously.

Feminists working outside the National Health Service can more easily develop alternative models, as Jane Black and Bie Nio Ong have done with their women's health courses and as Merryn Cooke describes in relation to the Rape Crisis Line. Those working within the NHS face the contradiction of being seen as aligning themselves with and at the same time criticising it and trying to build alternative ways of working. Whilst we value and are strongly committed to the NHS, we do not just want 'more of the same'. We do want more, but it must be very different from the often sexist and oppressive treatment meted out at present.

We face the contradiction, too, of being 'experts' and having a great deal of power over those who use our services. We may think we have clear ideas about what would be the best decision for our clients, and they may want us to decide for them. Should we do as they wish and take the decision, or should we try to help them to be self-determining? Whichever we decide, we are using our power over them and, as Carol Smith (1983) says, 'even big strong dykes want to be looked after sometimes!' What we try to do is to share our knowledge and skills with people so that they can take decisions for themselves. And if they then decide that they prefer a professional to take action on their behalf, they have made an informed choice.

'Vast spaces' (McRobbie 1982) like this may exist between feminist health workers and their clients, who are not used to exercising their own judgement about health care and are reluctant to overturn traditional professional–client relationships. But spaces of a different kind may be found when philosophies of life are widely divergent, as Bie Nio Ong has described in her work with women who abuse their children. Then it can be extremely difficult to understand the other point of view, and even harder to accept the limited possibility of sharing ideas and working together for change.

It can be very hard to work with other women who have no sympathy with a feminist approach to health care, or who do not see that women are oppressed and suffer in particular ways because they are women. Women nurses are an example of this, as Christine Webb discusses in relation to her research with gynaecological nurses. Nurses have traditionally functioned as advocates for doctors, and not for patients, and in colluding with the withholding of information, by covering up for doctors' omissions and inadequacies, and by protecting doctors from patients by 'gatekeeping', they have acted as 'token torturers' (Connors 1980). In striving to achieve 'professional status' for nursing, they have adopted a model of professionalism which sees the professional as an expert with a monopoly of knowledge and the patient as an ignorant object upon whom treatments are performed. Nurses thereby isolate themselves emotionally and socially both from their patients and from each other as women, and uphold the hostile beliefs about women which characterise our male-dominated society. If nurses were able to see themselves as women first, and then as nurses, they could 'begin to make meaningful connections with the lives of other nurses and women, establishing a community of shared caring' (Ashley 1980). They could then act as advocates for patients instead of doctors, and define a new kind of professionalism based on sharing knowledge, power and support, and on working for real health care for everyone and particularly for other women.

Feminist health care is an alternative form, but is very different from other so-called 'alternative' therapies which have grown in popularity in recent years. Homeopathy, acupuncture and other 'holistic' treatments frequently share the mystification and exploitative relationships found in 'scientific medicine'. Patients are treated as individuals by 'expert' practitioners who may be unwilling or unable to explain how the treatment is claimed to work, and who charge quite high fees for their work. If we demand that 'scientific medicine' gives us explanations and choices, then we must require the same of alternative medicine too, and not relax our standards simply because alternative practitioners spend more time with us and are more polite and caring in their attitudes than the professionals we are used to (Laws 1983; Smith 1983).

Feminist health care is based on quite different concepts. It sees people's health problems not as individual pathologies but as shared outcomes of the kind of society we live in. For women, this means acknowledging that sexist ideas and behaviour can make you sick, and therefore that in order to be healthy these ideas and behaviour must be changed. Sharing knowledge and power between practitioners and clients, breaking down the barriers of unequal relationships, and supporting people as they take decisions and make their own health choices are ways in which feminists work towards change.

We do not think that health care will be revolutionised overnight in this way, because its defects are problems for society as a whole and cannot be dealt with in individual health centres, hospital wards and clinics. But we do hope to cause ripples that may build up into bigger waves (McRobbie 1982). Or to use a perhaps more fitting analogy, we hope that by relieving some of the symptoms, we may become stronger and increase our resistance so that we can take care of others and ourselves and build a real health care service for everyone.

References

Ashley JA (1980) Power in structured misogyny implications for the politics of care. *Advances in Nursing Science,* **2** (3), 3–22
Connors DD (1980) Sickness unto death: medicine as mythic, necrophilic and iatrogenic. *Advances in Nursing Science,* **2** (3), 39–51
Laws S (1983) Women's health care and alternative medicine: reasons to believe? *Catcall,* **15**, 2–7
McRobbie A (1982) The politics of feminist research: between talk, text and action. *Feminist Review,* **12**, 46–57
Smith C (1983) Is alternative medicine necessarily better for women? *Catcall,* **15**, 8–14

Index

189